Health program evaluation

Issues and problems in health care

Paul R. Torrens, M.D., M.P.H., Series editor

School of Public Health,
University of California,
Los Angeles, California

Other available titles

Rural Health Care, Milton I. Roemer, M.D.
Elements of Planning for Area-Wide Personal Health Services,
   William Shonick, Ph.D.
The Law and the Public's Health, Kenneth R. Wing, J.D., M.P.H.
National Health Policy and the Underserved: Ethnic Minorities, Women,
   and the Elderly, Jerry L. Weaver, Ph.D.
The American Health Care System: Issues and Problems,
   Paul R. Torrens, M.D., M.P.H.

Forthcoming title

Issues in Women's Health Care, Helen I. Marieskind, Dr. P.H.

Health program evaluation

Stephen M. Shortell, Ph.D.
William C. Richardson, Ph.D.

Department of Health Services,
School of Public Health and Community Medicine,
University of Washington, Seattle, Washington

with 14 illustrations

The C. V. Mosby Company

Saint Louis   1978

The C. V. Mosby Company
11830 Westline Industrial Drive, St. Louis, Missouri 63141

Library of Congress Cataloging in Publication Data

Shortell, Stephen M.
  Health program evaluation.

  (Issues and problems in health care)
  Bibliography: p.
  1. Health services administration—Evaluation.
2. Public health—Evaluation. 3. Evaluation research
(Social action program) I. Richardson, William C.,
joint author. II. Title. [DNLM: 1. Health services
—United States. 2. Public health administration—
United States. 3. Evaluation studies. W84 AA1 S513h]
RA394.S56   362.1′04′25   78-4866
ISBN 0-8016-4595-6

C/M/M 9 8 7 6 5 4 3 2 1

For
Susan and Nancy
and our children
Stephanie, Juliana, Elizabeth, and Jennifer

Foreword

During the past decade, the cost for health care has been escalating at an alarming rate. In 1976, health care expenditures in the United States reached $139.3 billions, or 8.6 percent of the gross national product, compared to $4.2 billions or 5.8 percent ten years ago. As expenditures increased, the public sector's share rose from 25.7 percent of total expenditures in 1966 to 42.2 percent in 1976. This rapid increase has caused federal, state, and local officials to critically examine current and planned health care programs in order to make careful decisions about priorities and allocation of limited resources. Program evaluation is important to policymakers because it provides the sound factual basis for making these decisions. Whether we are determining how hospitals should be reimbursed or alternatives to institutional long-term care, program evaluation can provide a fresh, objective examination of the problems and issues involved. It can identify which programs are performing well or badly and why. Furthermore, program evaluation can furnish the data and information needed to strengthen weak programs, support effective programs, or eliminate programs that are not meeting legislative and/or agency goals and objectives. This feedback is extremely important to legislators and government officials.

Professors Stephen M. Shortell and William C. Richardson are to be commended for their interest in equipping present and future health service professionals for the task of dealing with questions of health program design, analysis, and evaluation. Their text underscores the compelling need for researchers to understand the political and administrative environment in which research and evaluation dealing with health service programs are likely to occur, since the nature of that milieu can contribute to the shape of the evaluation outcome. It attempts to bridge the two diverse worlds of the basic technical evaluation process on the one hand and, on the other, the political and administrative realities within which the assessment is conducted.

The authors have, to their credit, distinguished among various types of program settings and organizational issues that confound the evaluation process and that too often limit results despite the best design preparation and intention.

The Health Care Financing Administration (HCFA), one of the most recently created agencies of the Department of Health, Education, and Welfare, is especially concerned with effective health program evaluation through its Office of Policy, Planning, and Research. Since it assumed the combined responsibility for the administration of the Medicare and Medicaid programs, for professional standards review, and for research and statistics related to health care financing, its concerns have extended beyond the funding and management of a massive share of the nation's medical care services. The cost of health care, and its continuing escalation, impelled in part by new federal programs, requires that we attempt to test promising new proposals for improved financing, delivery, and organization of medical care before they reach the stage of legislative or operational readiness. Our ongoing experience must also be carefully examined for highlights leading to more effective management and public policy.

An increasing awareness of the evaluative function, however, pervades the entire health services structure so that administrators, program planners, and providers must be more directly concerned with the consequences of their actions as they seek to change health care organizations and improve medical care practices. Accountability by public officials as well as medical care providers is the inevitable consequence of growing consumer sophistication and public financing. Shortell and Richardson are keenly aware of this new responsibility that is being thrust upon us, and this text should prove a valuable resource for both current and future administrators, providers, and policymakers in meeting the challenge.

Robert A. Derzon

Administrator

Clifton R. Gaus

Associate Administrator for
Policy, Planning, and Research

Health Care Financing Administration,
Department of Health, Education, and Welfare

Foreword

For many of us, it is impossible to give up completely the stereotypes we hold about medical research and health care. The great medical discoveries of the 1800's, the magical control of tropical diseases during that century and the early decades of this one, and the prevention of communicable diseases by community-wide vaccination programs were truly remarkable demonstrations of human persistence and creativity. These events, reinforced by sometimes factually based and othertimes scientifically unsupported popular novels, and of course by the glamorization of practicing physicians and by the dramatization of the miracles of modern medical care on television, are responsible for the popular views on the power of medical research and the efficacy of health care.

It is important, however, that the stereotypes of medical research and health care not be accepted unquestioningly. As social medicine experts and medical historians have informed us repeatedly, most of the decisive reductions in mortality and morbidity are accounted for by improvements in general living conditions; moreover, as reviews of accomplishments in disease control report, new medical interventions and technological advances typically result in only marginal improvements in health status. Certainly now, except for a few disease areas and in some underdeveloped countries, reduction of morbidity and mortality is an incremental, not a revolutionary, process. Further, increasingly, the chief architects of improved health status and the important warriors against illness and disease are the specialists identified with community medicine, public health and the delivery of health services.

Surely, there will be additional laboratory achievements in medicine and more technological breakthroughs in diagnosis and treatment. But it is a safe prediction that future improvements in the health and comfort of community members, even more than in the past, will be accomplished by attacking the defective conditions of our social milieu and physical environment, by remedying the personal and interpersonal behaviors of community members so that prevention and compliance increase, and by reorganizing the delivery of health services so that access to and continuity of competent health care is universally available. It is these areas that are emphasized in current health initiatives to expand and restructure inner city ambulatory care and increase the number of competence of rural health providers, in the emergence of a variety of new health practitioners, in the revitalization of health education, in attacks on industrial and environmental pollution, in the expansion of mental health activities, and in the press for expanded governmental support of the costs of health care.

In some areas, the efforts of the last decade are impressive, as in the markedly increased access to care of the urban poor and minority group members. In others it is disheartening, as in the cases of tobacco smoking, drug addition, obesity, and many other health-threatening behaviors. Moreover, some of the efforts that have proved successful in terms of their objectives have been accompanied by fearsome side effects, including the spiraling of costs of health services and consumer disenchantment with the health care system. Economic resource constraints as well as the power of social traditions and cultural norms, not to mention the rigidities of extant bureaucratic arrangements and the self-interests of various parties within the health industry, impede efforts directed at the goal of improved health status for community members. The dictum that gains in the health field usually are incremental and modest and that many initiatives and innovative programs are, on balance, either ineffective or inefficient, must be accepted now as in the past, despite our romantic stereotypes of progress in medical care and health status.

Rather than to "eyeball" the effects of programs and initiatives in public health and medical care, and to depend on judgmental impressions of the utility of different delivery of health services approaches, it is essential that as systematic, replicable, and precise assessments as possible be undertaken of both established and innovative efforts. Unless the press is toward such assessments, modest gains may be overlooked and either ineffective or overly costly interventions adopted, with consequent loss of support by disgruntled influentials and political and community groups.

Besides, data, evidence, and the rigor of scientific inquiry have characterized the adoption of new procedures and practices in the health area since the beginnings of modern medicine. That "proof" needs to be obtained by a set of rules is not disagreeable either to the laboratory scientist or the clinical investigator, and it should not be for the health professional engaged in the innovation and conduct of macro-activities. This is all evaluation research is, a set of procedures that when properly implemented allow inference, with as much certainty as possible, to be drawn about the feasibility, efficacy, and efficiency of various approaches to the prevention, control, and management of disease and the organization and arrangement for the delivery of health services.

Evaluation research, in a sense, is an organizing concept. In its basic perspective, it makes use, as much of this text indicates, in the underlying commitment to the "experiment," to the basic outlook of the laboratory scientist. In its data collection approach, as other parts document, its procedures often are the same as those employed by the epidemiologist. The practicing professional, the health science student, and the medical investigator, then, will feel comfortable with much of the material included here. The chapters, in this perspective, represent a codification and a restatement of how to accumulate evidence, how to make inferences and how to utilize research for health care interventions.

At the same time, the volume contains much new material for the health professional and researcher, for evaluation research is rooted to a large extent in social research methodologies. Moreover, evaluation research, as an outlook and a set of procedures, is equally commonplace in welfare, education, and public safety efforts—indeed, across the entire human services arena—as in the health field. Many of the ideas, principles, and techniques presented are drawn from the accumulating body of evaluation research being undertaken in different fields. The authors have strived, however, to create a text about health evaluations and have employed and adopted examples and illustrations to meet the objective of providing a special book for the field.

To my knowledge, this is the first basic text on *health* evaluations. Not only does its specialized character make instruction in evaluation research more relevant to persons in the health field, but it brings together for the professional and investigator procedures and viewpoints previously scattered in the elusive and varied evaluation research literature. The authors have also strived to make the book short without sacrificing completeness, and readable without being over-simple.

One final observation: the successful conduct of evaluation research requires attention to practical as well as technical details. Evaluations are exciting but difficult to do well because of the contingencies that surround doing research in the complex community and organizational world in which health care activities are lodged. Many of the pages of this text provide advice in these practical matters —the section on how to state program objectives is but one example. Readers of this text, in undertaking their own evaluations, and in appreciating the results of work done by others, I am certain, will come to appreciate the effort to consider both the technical and pragmatic elements involved in evaluation research.

Howard E. Freeman

Institute for Social Science Research,
University of California,
Los Angeles, Calif.

Preface

Over the past several years, we have been teaching program evaluation to graduate students interested in the administration and delivery of health services. A major difficulty in teaching this material involves the wide variation in students' academic backgrounds, resulting in problems of what to include and exclude and at what level to present the material. The problem is complicated by an evaluation literature scattered throughout widely different sources. For a discussion of experimental and quasi-experimental designs, one draws on Campbell and Stanley *(Experimental and Quasi-Experimental Designs for Research);* for discussion of measurement reliability and validity issues, the educational psychology literature is helpful; for discussion of evaluation design in health services, Suchman *(Evaluation Research: Principles and Practice in Public Service and Social Action Programs)* is a useful source; for empirical examples, several collections of readings are available (for example, Caro, *Readings in Evaluation Research;* Schulberg and others, *Program Evaluation in the Health Fields;* Mullen, *Evaluation of Social Intervention;* and Struening and Guttentag, *Handbook of Evaluation Research, Volume II).* One goes to still other sources for discussion of program implementation (for example, Williams and Elmore, *Social Program Implementation),* the administrative and political issues surrounding program evaluation (for example, Weiss, *Evaluation Research),* and the role of program evaluation in the development and implementation of public policy.

To a great extent this diversity reflects an increased interest in program evaluation itself, and it should be applauded. It is up to the instructor to integrate the material in a way that contributes to the learning objectives of the students. But we believe the process can be expedited by developing course material that brings together "in one place" some of the key concepts, methodologies, and issues related to program evaluation in general and their applications to the delivery of health services in particular.

The major purpose of this textbook, then, is to provide a systematic presentation of the major concepts, methodologies, and issues concerning the evaluation of health services delivery programs at a level appropriate to graduate students in health services administration and planning, public health, dentistry, medicine, nursing, pharmacy, social work, and related health professions. As Henderson and Meinert note: "Most of the textbooks in the fields of both epidemiology and biostatistics devote little space to design and analysis questions related to health and medical evaluation." This book is thus aimed primarily at individuals who will eventually be involved in the administration, planning, delivery, and evaluation of health services programs. The text will also be a useful first source to discipline-oriented students (for example, in psychology, sociology, education) or others who wish to specialize and become "experts" in evaluation research itself. For such students, however, the material in this text would need to be supplemented by additional readings and coursework.

This book also attempts to redress an imbalance caused by the somewhat artificial distinction between technical/methodological evaluation issues and the political and administrative settings in which evaluation is conducted. It is our belief that the future administrator, planner, or provider of health services needs to know something about both evaluation research itself and the environment in which it takes place. For us, the relevant question is not should future administrators, planners, and providers be trained to do research, but rather, what does an understanding of the evaluation research process contribute to their overall competence and effectiveness? It is hoped that the sensitivity of the health science student to the importance of program evaluation will be increased, together with a further understanding of the uses and limitations of program evaluation in the decision-making and policy-making processes.

The contents of the book are organized in a sequence that we have found useful in communicating with students. However, the individual chapters are sufficiently self-contained that other instructors can use the material in a different order or can assign specific chapters at different points in the course. The first chapter traces some of the early background and historical development of program evaluation efforts in the health care field and describes some contemporary forces influencing the current shape and content of health program evaluations. In Chapter 2, the student is introduced to issues concerning the development of program objectives, different levels and types of objectives, and the design of program components. In Chapter 3, some major experimental and quasi-experimental designs applicable to health program evaluation are discussed. Emphasis is placed on the pros and cons of each design relevant to issues of internal and external validity. Chapter 4 then builds on Chapter 3 by discussing issues related to the reliability and validity of individual measures, the advantages and disadvantages of different methods of data collection, and basic data analysis approaches. In Chapter 5, the important administrative and political issues in program evaluation are discussed, along with an analysis of the problems of program evaluation. Chapter 6 concludes with a discussion of future issues in program evaluation, with an emphasis on the role of program evaluation in developing and implementing public policy in the delivery of health services.

At the end of each chapter, where pertinent, a glossary of terms is presented, along with class problem exercises and a list of suggested readings. In addition an Appendix presents an example of a student's evaluation research paper. We have found the problem exercises, together with the requirement that a student develop an evaluation of an ongoing delivery program, to be valuable learning experiences that reinforce the course readings and classroom discussions.

From the preceding comments and, hopefully, from the material to follow, it may appear that this book represents a rational approach to the subject. However, it was not written in a particularly rational environment. Contrary to what may prevail elsewhere, and certainly contrary to common opinion, this book was not written in the quiet solitude of an academic leave of absence, sabbatical, or even an "off quarter" from teaching, research, or administrative responsibilities. Rather, it was written in hotel rooms, on airplanes, in airports, on buses, between classes and student counseling sessions, between faculty meetings, and, yes, *in* faculty meetings! Thus, whatever clarity and coherence may exist in the chapters that follow are due in small part to our perseverance and in large part to the skill and careful attention of our editor, Augie Podolinsky, the secretarial support provided by Bernice Goldberg and Elaine Morrisey, and the library research provided by Diane McKenzie. The book has also benefited greatly from the comments and suggestions of our colleagues at the University of Washington—Allan Blackman, Marilyn Bergner, and Walt Williams—and, in particular, from the advice of Ron Andersen, University of Chicago, and Don Riedel, presently University of Washington and formerly Yale University. It is entirely possible that a key point raised by them has been lost somewhere along the way (perhaps at an airport terminal), but as teachers of program planning and evaluation in their own right, they will be able to remedy our neglect or shortcomings. This, of course, applies to all future users of this text.

Finally, as implied already, this text represents a beginning. Since the ultimate test of program evaluation itself is the extent to which it is actually used by, and is useful to, those who have to make program decisions, so too the merit of this text must be judged by those who find it useful in teaching program evaluation to health science students. The ultimate impact, of course, must be judged by the increasing numbers of health science students (administrators, planners, direct providers) who have an understanding and a working knowledge of program evaluation methodologies and who can carry this over into their professional practice. We are, of course, not so optimistic or naive to think that this in itself will have an impact on the health status of the United States population. Rather, we hope it may help everyone (administrator, planner, provider, and consumer) to better understand the uses and limits of health service in a complex society.

Stephen M. Shortell

William C. Richardson

Someone has suggested that evaluation is like salt.
Some foods need more salt than others,
but too much salt can ruin a meal.

A. L. Knudson,

"Evaluation for What?"

Dogma is the enemy of truth and the enemy of persons.
The ideas enshrined in dogma may include good and wise ideas,
but dogma is bad in itself because it is accepted
as good without examination.

OK Words

Contents

CHAPTER 1

Program evaluation: historical antecedents and contemporary developments

The purpose of this chapter is to introduce students and practitioners in the health sciences to some basic developments in the evolution of program evaluation. A *program* is defined here as ". . . an organized response to eliminate or reduce one or more problems where the response includes one or more objectives, performance of one or more activities, and expenditure of resources."[1]

A number of terms will be defined and compared. These include (1) evaluation research, (2) nonevaluative research, (3) policy research, (4) policy analysis, (5) impact or "summative" evaluation, and (6) process or "formative" evaluation. Factors shaping both the growth and nature of future program evaluation will also be explored. The many motivations for conducting program evaluation activities will be discussed. Finally, the relevance of program evaluation for practicing administrators, planners, and providers will be noted. Comprehension of the material in this chapter provides a framework for understanding future chapters and will enhance the reader's eventual ability to analyze, apply, synthesize, and evaluate what is to be learned from this text.

Historical development

Attempting to evaluate a social program is at best risky and at worst treacherous. In few other activities are the ambivalent tendencies of society so clearly revealed. On the one hand is society's desire to learn more so that the quality of life may be improved, while on the other hand is the ubiquitous fear of what might be found. It is a phenomenon similar to individual growth and development, but it is acted out and institutionalized at the level of social collectives with consequences that frequently have far-reaching implications for large numbers of people. This tug-of-war between the desire to learn more and the need for self-protection is frequently the genesis of social conflict and social change, and is clearly revealed as one traces the evolution of health services over the past several centuries. A brief review of this evolution is important *not* because history might repeat itself, but because what is learned from previous experiences, with adaptation, may be applicable in present circumstances.

Evaluation of medical care services has existed in some form from earliest times. We know that such evaluations were often closely tied to sanctions. For

1

example, in 3000 BC Egypt, if the patient were to unnecessarily lose an eye, the physician was subject to the loss of a hand![2] Similar sanctions were meted out for less than adequate outcomes involving other bodily parts. Of course, we are not told what criteria were used in the determination of "unnecessary," a problem that continues to plague program evaluation of quality of medical care up to the present.

Prior to the eighteenth century, there was little in the way of *formal* evaluation of health and social services. As Suchman notes, with the development of the period of revolution and enlightenment in the eighteenth century came the first major thrust of experimentation and evaluation of public service programs, and these activities have accelerated in recent times.[3]

Three primary reasons can be cited for this development. The first concerns the general increase in the complexity of social life. With complexity comes a search for answers to how society's activities of daily living might better be conducted. Second, investigative tools are needed to provide information. The major breakthrough in the eighteenth and nineteenth centuries provided the scientific arsenal necessary to the task. Third is the dramatic growth of service industries, especially governmentally financed services in almost every society. These services cannot be evaluated solely by market mechanisms.

Together, these three factors (increased complexity of life, available scientific methodology, and the growth of service industries) acted as a catalyst for more formal inquiry into the evaluation of public health programs. Vital statistics and morbidity and mortality data were first proposed as early as 1662[3]; pioneers such as Lemuel Shattuck, Edwin Chadwick, and C.E.A. Winslow were strong early proponents for the systematic collection of such data to evaluate the effectiveness of community health programs. Interest in evaluation gradually grew, but not with the same intensity as interest in providing services, particularly in areas of obvious need. As Suchman notes, "So great was the faith in service techniques that public agency and community workers usually begrudged any diversion of effort or funds away from them. For example, where the handicapped children's programs achieved nationwide attention, the cry was for more clinics, more children brought to care, more programs offering corrective services. Not one carefully planned, controlled, prospective evaluation study of the long-range restorative power of these programs was conducted."[3] The same statement can be applied to a number of new health care delivery programs in more recent times.

Following World War I, as programs continued to expand, interest grew in evaluating the effort or processes of service delivery. This commonly took the form of self-rating appraisals. They were seriously deficient in their (1) neglect of outcome measures of program effectiveness; (2) use of objectives based on untested, unstated, and frequently erroneous assumptions; (3) reliance on biased data and samples of unknown representation; (4) failure to follow principles of sound experimental design; (5) inadequate attention given to the accuracy, reliability, and validity of measurement; and, therefore, (6) inability to draw causal inferences regarding program effects, which contributed little to the advancement of knowledge regarding the programs under study.[3]

In recent times, and in particular since the mid-1960s, explicit attempts have been made to remedy many of these shortcomings. Critical to this development has been the increased training of both those who are usually the doers of evaluation (academically trained if not academically based social scientists) and those who are the facilitators and users of evaluation (program administrators and planners, agency officials, and direct providers of care). There are few who believe that such training alone will lead to better conceived and more useful program evaluations, but also few who believe that such evaluations will come about without such exposure. For example, a recent study of five groups of health care experts revealed unanimous agreement that a major barrier to improving the quality of health services is a lack of "evaluation skills of providers for proposed innovations."[4] In brief, better and broader-based training is a necessary but not sufficient condition for better program evaluations.

A number of observers, most notably Weiss[5] and Williams,[6] suggest that more rigorous methodological tools and designs focusing on impact or outcome evaluations may not be the solution to better program evaluation. Impact or outcome evaluations are sometimes referred to as *summative* evaluations. Rather, what is needed is a better understanding of specific program components and the process by which they are implemented. Such evaluations are sometimes referred to as *formative* evaluations. Many programs fail because they never get to the stage of being evaluated based on their outcomes and yet, with few exceptions,[7] little is known about the causes of such failures. This concern with how programs get put into place has come to be called "implementation assessment"[6] and is particularly relevant to large-scale social experiments. The advocates of implementation assessments do not deny the advantages of soundly designed outcome evaluations of program effects but, rather, remind us that before its effects or impacts can be studied the first question that must be asked is whether the program is operational.

A related issue concerns the process by which soundly executed process and outcome evaluations of programs found to be successful may be spread to other agencies and groups in society. For example, Henderson and Meinert note that randomized clinical trials have had limited impact on the actual practice of medicine, due largely to inadequate understanding of or attention to implementation, social change, and diffusion issues involved in the delivery of medical services in action settings.[8]

The interplay between implementation and outcome assessments (between formative and summative evaluation) will become an increasingly important issue in the evaluation of health services programs. This issue takes on considerable national significance when it is noted that of the $75 million spent on evaluation research in 1975, 38 percent was for evaluation of health care delivery programs of one form or another.[9] A number of forces shaping this development deserve comment.

Contemporary forces
New federal programs

Beginning with the Kennedy and Johnson administrations, the number of new federal programs concerned with health services has grown tremendously. These programs gave birth to many new delivery organizations, including neighborhood health centers, regional medical programs, comprehensive health planning agencies, and experimental health services delivery systems, to mention only a few. These coupled with the introduction of Medicare (Title XVIII) and Medicaid (Title XIX) represent expanding efforts by the federal government to intervene directly into the delivery and organization of health care services. Early experience with many of these programs led to the realization of the need for cost and quality control and the need for rigorous evaluation of program effects. But as Bice and associates have noted, "One seeks in vain, however, for findings from evaluation studies that offer clear-cut directions to policy-makers. Although aspects of each program have been studied by various investigators, none can estimate unequivocally their impacts on the health of populations, isolate their unique contribution to the organization and delivery of health services, or even describe coherently and concisely what local organizations do and have done. This state of affairs, we suggest, is due to several conceptual and methodological issues that have not been satisfactorily resolved by social scientists concerned with the study of organizations and political processes, as well as to fundamental ambiguities built into such programs."[10]

These observations highlight the fact that the evaluation of many of the newer health care programs is not simply a matter of better measurement and better experimental designs but also a matter of studying the organizational and political processes within which programs are developed and implemented. If anything, new developments concerned with Health Systems Agencies (HSAs), Professional Standards Review Organizations (PSROs), and rate review groups further emphasize the importance of taking into account organizational and political processes.

Budget pressures

While many programs have been designed to increase access to medical care or provide more "appropriate" forms of treatment, they have also resulted in increased expenditures for health services. In 1976, health services accounted for 8.7 percent of the gross national product (GNP) versus 5.9 percent in 1965 and 4.1 percent in 1940.[11] Thus, great pressure has been placed on program administrators at all levels to contain costs and to justify the cost-effectiveness of current operations. A growing percentage of federally awarded programmatic support has built-in evaluation requirements (for example, Community Mental Health Center Act).

New technology

A third important development leading to greater emphasis on evaluation research has been the continued growth of medical science and technology and its application to the delivery of personal health care services. New diagnostic tools (such as CAT scanners) and therapeutic methodologies (for example, coronary bypass surgery, renal dialysis) have alerted many observers to call for rigorous evaluation of the cost-benefit, or at least cost-effectiveness, of such new technologies. Brook notes, "A lot of technology that has been implemented in this country has not been evaluated in any way, shape or form, whether by randomized clinical trials, by time series analysis, or anything. They just have not been evaluated. The argument could be made that we need to develop a policy that would require rigorous evaluation of new technologies before they are disseminated."[12] To what extent does the new technology replace existing technology, complement existing technology, or even lead to new uses of existing technology? What are the effects on the decision-making process in health care delivery? These issues frequently assume greater importance as a result of ethical concerns regarding the extension and quality of life associated with the use of new technology.

Emphasis on preventive care

Because of both the increased cost of medical care and the sometimes disappointing results, a growing interest has developed in preventive care. While preventive care is a broad concept covering a multitude of behaviors, its advocates assert that by diagnosing and treating illness in the early stages, a significant amount of money can be saved while increasing the probability of successfully restoring the patient to good health. The issue of the potential efficacy of preventive care is, of course, much more complex, requiring conceptualization of those specific conditions and socioeconomic characteristics of patients for whom preventive care might have some impact. For example, while there are clear advantages to immunization of children, little is known about the circumstances under which annual physical examinations or various screening programs, such as Pap smears to detect cancer of the cervix, are effective. Again, the issue of evaluation of preventive care programs is not only an issue of more methodologically rigorous evaluation but also one of organization and politics of health care consumer and provider groups.

Public accountability

For a variety of reasons—moral, legal, financial, and educational—the public is demanding that service organizations of all sorts, not just health, be more explicitly accountable for the form and quality of services delivered. Since this trend is not likely to be reversed in the near future, if ever, it represents another major pressure on the administrator to formally evaluate program operations.

Increased professional conflict

As health care services have become more complex with the development of new technology, they have also become fragmented in their delivery by a variety of highly trained medical specialists. This has given rise to pleas for more coordinated approaches to patient care, such as health care teams. This development, in turn, represents another area for systematic evaluation. For example, it is somewhat ironic to note that the introduction of new health practitioners (physician assistants, nurse practitioners), designed to increase physician productivity and perhaps contain costs, also adds more types of providers to the vast array already available to the health care consumer. It also places a great strain on established professional identities and role relationships as attempts are made to incorporate these new health practitioners into traditional practice settings. Available evidence indicates that even when new organizations are developed to make use of new forms of health manpower, significant problems occur.[13] This suggests that not only does the introduction of new health practitioners require more formal evaluation but, at the same time, the development itself with its attendant conflict among professionals will make such evaluations difficult to execute. As with other programs, evaluation may best begin by simply documenting the implementation process, the problems that occurred, and the strategies used in dealing with them.

Interdependence of problems

The problems associated with delivering health care are not isolated ones. However, many of the new federal as well as nonfederal programs were developed as if the issues and problems were quite unrelated to one another (for example, the Medicaid experience in most states regarding access and cost tradeoffs). Issues of access, cost, quality, comprehensiveness, and continuity of care, to mention a few, are interconnected, and great demand will be placed on program administrators and evaluators to provide for such complexity. This means not only more sophisticated evaluation designs but also greater attention to the tradeoffs and side payments made by the various actors involved in implementing specific programs.

Large-scale interventions

Given the growing importance of the decisions facing policy-makers in the health care arena and the increased complexity and interdependence of the issues, a tendency is developing to fund more large-scale demonstration experiments. The emphasis on demonstrations is consistent with the American philosophy of incrementalism in political decision-making and, to some extent, is inherent in democratic systems. Examples of large-scale intervention in health services include hospital prospective reimbursement experiments and the experimental health services delivery systems, but undoubtedly the prime example is the Rand Health Insurance Experiment.[14] In this study the price and scope of benefits of insurance packages are experimentally varied, and then attempts are made to assess the impact on use, cost, and quality of care provided. While a great deal of controversy surrounds such expensive, large-scale experiments, indications are that they are not likely to go away. Program administrators and providers are likely to become more involved in such large-scale interventions, where the implications extend beyond their immediate personal and organizational interests.

The rise of administration

A final force shaping the growth and nature of evaluation of health services is the growth of administration itself. The increased complexity of organization and issues has brought a great demand for trained administrative personnel. Perrow has traced the relative power shifts among medical staff, trustees, and administrative groups in hospitals over the years and has shown the net relative gain accruing to administrators.[15] The tremendous growth in the number of graduate programs in health services administration, from approximately eleven accredited programs in 1952 to thirty-six in 1976, and in the number of graduates per year, from approximately 177 in 1952 to 1,053 in 1976, attests to the growing importance of administration.[16, 17]

A major attribute of administrative theory is its emphasis on *rational* decision-making. While there are many constraints on rational decision-making in practice, it would seem that the growth of professional health services administration has contributed to a more systematic scrutiny of allocation decisions in health care organizations and has provided some motivation for attempts to formally evaluate key programs. This, of course, is more true in recent years with the development of incentives (or sanctions) for better performance in the cost and quality areas of service delivery.

These factors are believed to be the most important forces influencing the growing demand for formal evaluation of health services programs and shaping the nature of the evaluative process. They are *likely to prevail for many years* and, thus, represent factors that must be dealt with by the administrators, planners, and providers of tomorrow. The common thread running through all is the emphasis on *rationalizing* the delivery of services. That is, the emphasis is not only on whether the program worked (improved access, contained costs) but on *why* the effort was brought about (or not brought about, as the case may be). And the questions of *why* and *how* include paying attention to the issues surrounding program implementation. As will become clearer in subsequent chapters, the emphasis on *rationality* becomes the key link between the administrative and clinical aspects of service delivery and the evaluation of these services. And it is for this reason, as indicated in the preface, that program evaluation is an increasingly important area of study for future health services administrators, planners, and providers. To pinpoint this relevance more clearly, one must define precisely what is meant by evaluation research and, in particular, program evaluation.

What is evaluation research?
Evaluative versus nonevaluative research

To the extent that *judgment* is involved in decision-making, evaluation is taking place. In this respect, administrators, planners, and providers are being involved in evaluational activities on a daily basis. The decisions to hire or fire an employee, to expand facilities, to initiate a new program are all *evaluative* decisions. But what distinguishes program *evaluation research* from day-to-day evaluative decisions is the use of the *scientific method*. The essence of the scientific method is the attempt to isolate causes of particular events or outcomes. If a particular program appears to be associated with a beneficial effect, one must know whether the effects can really be attributable to the program or whether they might result from some other factor. Program evaluation, of course, is not unique in the use of the scientific method to arrive at judgments. Rather, the scientific method and its approximations are at the core of most basic or *nonevaluative* research designed to contribute to disciplinary knowledge in, for example, economics, sociology, or psychology. The primary distinction, then, between program evaluation and basic or nonevaluative research lies not in the methods used but rather in the uses of the knowledge acquired. In program evaluation the emphasis is on judging the worth of a specific program or project whose results are to be used by program administrators, planners, and providers of services to improve, extend, or in some way modify (including the possibility of doing away with) the program. In contrast, the primary goal of nonevaluative research is to contribute to disciplinary knowledge and understanding of social and physical phenomena that may or may not be directly useful, particularly in the short run, to those charged with operating programs and providing services.

An example may serve to clarify the distinction between evaluative and nonevaluative research. Let us suppose that a hospital develops a continuing education program for physicians on the management of hypertension. An attempt to evaluate the impact of this program on the physicians' knowledge and behavior or, indeed, on outcomes (perhaps measured by a patient's age-adjusted blood pressure) to see whether the program had an effect and how it might be improved would serve as an example of program evaluation research.

In contrast, the physician continuing education program could be used as a setting by behavioral scientists to test various theories of motivation and learning associated with the educational process—this is an example of nonevaluative basic science research. While this example serves to clarify the distinction between the two forms of research, the distinction is frequently overdrawn, with particularly serious consequences for the quality and reliability of program evaluations. Simply put, it is difficult to answer the questions of *how* and *why* a program worked or did not work without having some underlying *theory* of *how and why* the program was supposed to bring about certain expected changes. For example, how can one understand the impact of a continuing education program for physicians without having some knowledge of the underlying learning and motivational characteristics of the educational process for the group involved? Or, how can a hospital administrator really make the most use of findings which suggest that special nurse-mother interactions reduce the stress experienced by children having tonsillectomies unless he has some understanding of a theory of stress and the particular components of a new program that appear to affect levels of stress?

This is particularly true when, as is frequently the case, the outcome measures indicate no change, or only slight beneficial effects. In such situations, the obvious administrative question to ask is *why* the results were less than desired or expected, *what* can be done to improve the program, and *how* should such changes take place? Without a clearly specified theory of *how* and *why* "x" and what specific components of "x" were supposed to produce "y," the administrator is left to consider these questions in a vacuum.

There is, then, a need for sound theoretical thinking in the design of applied program evaluations, and this situation suggests opportunities for mutual collaboration between academic and nonacademic-based social scientists on the one hand and program administrators and providers on the other. From the perspective of the academic program evaluator, it also suggests the possibility that one can contribute useful information to program administrators and providers who have to make operational decisions as well as contribute to the advancement of disciplinary knowledge regarding particular theories of social phenomena. This, of course, is not easily achieved; the tensions inherent in the differing perspectives of the administrator/planner/ provider and the disciplinary evaluator are discussed fully in Chapter 5. But it is important for the reader to recognize the bridge between evaluative and nonevaluative research, a bridge that is based not solely on the uses of the scientific method (or approximations to it) in research design, but rather on the importance of theory to the administrator/planner/provider charged with making decisions or changes regarding operating programs. One should also recognize the importance of health delivery program settings to the academic evaluator interested in advancing disciplinary knowledge as well as contributing useful information for program decision-making.

Policy research versus policy analysis

Two other terms require definition as well, *policy research* and *policy analysis*. *Policy research* in health services refers to investigations directed toward specific problems associated with the delivery of health services, the results of which are needed by or intended to be useful to individuals and groups who may make decisions or may be affected by decisions regarding the specific problems in question. Such research would include most program evaluation research efforts but would not be limited to them. Neither would policy research be limited to producing quick, short-run information. Rather, it would also encompass research designed to increase our understanding and knowledge of health services delivery, which may take several years to produce but which will, in the long run, inform public policy options regarding health care delivery. Thus, policy research is defined quite broadly to include not only specific program evaluations but also descriptive analyses of issues, nonexperimental cross-sectional analyses, and basic research designed to improve measurement of key analytical variables such as access to care, continuity of care, or quality of care. While program evaluation may *generally* be considered a subset of policy research, it is *not* the case that all program evaluations automatically serve as examples of policy research. The policy relevance of program evaluations depends on three factors: (1) the importance of the questions being addressed, (2) the extent to which user groups have been identified, and (3) the extent to which the results can be generalized to other situations and settings (external validity). As will be discussed in the following section, program evaluations are carried on for a number of reasons, sometimes having little to do with developing program or policy options. For example, a program may be evaluated as a "whitewash" job if the evaluation is designed to "fit" a foregone conclusion.

Health policy analysis involves the drawing together and evaluation of existing research, information, and informed judgment regarding the implications of alternative strategies for dealing with a specific problem or set of problems associated with the delivery of health services. It attempts to articulate and provide evidence for the pros and cons of alternative options or strategies facing a decision-maker in the health arena. Seldom will policy analysis be based on a single program evaluation but rather on a synthesis of programmatic evaluation as well as a review of relevant nonexperimental research and informed judgment on the issue. A *common* feature of both policy research and policy analysis is the identification of constituent groups interested in using the results of the research and analysis. This is perhaps most apparent and well-defined in the use of policy analyis and usually less defined, but of no lesser importance, in policy research. The prototypical relationships among program evaluation, nonevaluative research, policy research, and policy analysis are shown in Fig. 1, along with a specific example of each.

Examples of terms used in Fig. 1

1. *nonevaluative research* An investigation of role conflict among health care professionals to test and refine existing theories of role conflict. While such research may "by chance" be useful to administrators and providers, no explicit attempts are made to ensure such usefulness.
2. *nonevaluative policy research* Methodological research to develop better measure of health status to be used eventually by administrators, planners, providers, and policy-makers in the development, implementation, and evaluation of health care programs.
3. *evaluative research* After-the-fact evaluations of the cost-effectiveness and cost-benefits of coronary care units where there is little or no opportunity for such information to influence public policy regarding whether such units should have been built.

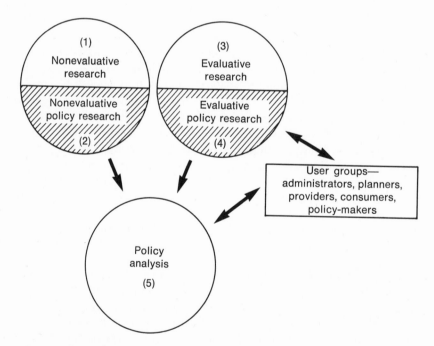

Fig. 1. Types of research and analysis. The double-headed arrows indicate that user groups contribute to the research and analysis process (particularly in the definition of issues) as well as using the results obtained.

4. *evaluative policy research* Evaluation of the effects of methadone maintenance programs on the rehabilitation of drug addicts. Evaluation of the effects of different benefit structures and copayment arrangements on demand for medical care.
5. *policy analysis* Examination of the existing evidence regarding the impact of certificate-of-need legislation in the light of alternative policies for regulating hospital costs.

Why evaluate?

The need for individuals and groups to seek yardsticks for evaluating performance and the factors associated with the growing demand for evaluation have been described and would seem to provide a natural answer to the question, "Why evaluate?" But as in most issues surrounding program evaluation, the answer is not so obvious. The question becomes more complex if one poses the question in a different form, namely, "From whose viewpoint?" This is the first important question to consider in program evaluation, even prior to asking what is to be evaluated and specifying measurable objectives.

There are at least five generic viewpoints to be considered in addressing this issue. These are the viewpoints of the organization, the individual program administrator, the funding agency, the public, and the program evaluator.[18] The *organization's* interest in evaluation may be to:

1. Demonstrate to other groups that the program is "effective"
2. Justify past or projected expenditures
3. Determine costs
4. Gain support for expansion of facilities, equipment, or programmatic activities
5. Satisfy funding agencies demanding evidence for program effects
6. Determine future courses of action

Individual program administrators will add their own agenda. They may view the evaluation as:

1. Bringing favorable attention to the particular unit or program
2. Providing a means of increasing one's status in the organization
3. Providing a means toward promotion
4. Being simply the "in" thing to do
5. Providing a means of gaining greater program control
6. Providing evidence to support a proposal for more program support

The *funding agency's* motives may center on:

1. The need to know the efficiency of program operation
2. The need to know the impact of effectiveness of the program
3. The need to demonstrate programmatic impact in a political context

From the viewpoint of the *public* and *consumer groups*, the primary motivations may be:

1. The efficiency with which tax dollars are spent
2. An interest in learning about the specific benefits provided—issues of accountability
3. A need to learn more about the value of planned change
4. An opportunity for increased community participation in social programs

Finally, one must consider the views of the *program evaluators* themselves. These may include:

1. The desire to contribute to disciplinary and applied knowledge
2. An opportunity for professional advancement
3. A sympathy with the program's goals
4. A strong belief in the importance of sound evaluation to make progress toward agency and societal goals

These viewpoints are meant to serve only as examples and are not exhaustive. Rather, they draw attention to the issue that for any single evaluative study the goals, aims, or motivations of the various parties involved are not likely to be in accord. The administrator of an outreach program for a neighborhood health center may view the proposed program evaluation quite differently from the way the president of the board of directors might view it, and their views may differ from those of the federal agencies involved, the program evaluation team, and the clients being served. These groups may agree on certain basic objectives—a sufficient base upon which to proceed with a sound evaluation—but each will also have its own latent objectives and hidden agendas which, as will be described in Chapter 5, will challenge the most conscientious and creative evaluator.

Agency officials, administrators, and providers should be particularly sensitive to the potential usefulness of program evaluations. Not only will such evaluations be required by federal and other granting agencies, but they can serve as a basic management tool for evaluating performance. This is particularly true in the case of (1) major new programs, such as inpatient versus outpatient treatment of alcoholism, (2) major changes in existing services, such as from team nursing to primary care nursing, and (3) high-risk decisions when time is available to accumulate data before the decision, such as whether to treat alcoholics in a separate unit or with other hospital patients. Evaluation assists the agency administrator or provider in answering the fundamental question: "Is the program doing any good?" The answer to this question (and, as we shall see in subsequent chapters, it is not usually a simple answer) provides input into the next sequence of decision-making concerning the allocation of the organization's resources for different programs and activities. Program evaluation can also serve as a primary source of accountability to oneself and one's staff, in addition to the clients being served. It serves to remind the organization and those involved in the program to be *results-oriented*. Too frequently, programs become so oriented toward the implementation of means that the original goals and objectives are obscured. Formal program evaluations based on clearly stated and measurable objectives force those involved to keep the end-state goals clearly in view. Further, the very process of thinking through a formal evaluation of a program contributes to the development of rigorous analytical thinking on the part of program managers and providers, with the effects carrying over into other organizational activities.

Although seldom mentioned, program evaluations can play a role in training staff and, by this process, introducing change into the organization. McCullough notes: "If the administrator does not see the usefulness of data to management, he will not see the usefulness of providing training to his evaluation staff. Without his support, nothing happens. In the same way as evaluative data can be used as a stimulus for change in mental health services, training can easily be conceptualized as a vehicle for organizational change."[19]

Finally, interest in formal program evaluation may be viewed as the *sine qua non* of professional practice and outlook. Again, McCullough notes: "The individual professions need to continue their efforts to pass along ethical and performance standards and to teach laboratory research techniques. But, they also need to lay the groundwork in their students for judging the effects of programs and of judging their impact on social problems. It is unreasonable to tell students they must do program evaluation or to exhort working professionals to do the same without giving them *some* information about what to do and how to do it. That is, training in techniques and methods is needed but a major issue is still that it is the individual who is responsible for not only maintaining professional standards but also for evaluating his efforts and for utilizing the results. It is that interest and/or motivation that professional education should build into its students."[19]

Summary

In summary, from the administrator, planner, and provider perspective, program evaluation helps to answer basic questions concerning whether the program is any good; helps ensure accountability to oneself, one's staff, and one's clients; helps to keep the emphasis on end-results; contributes to the development of analytical processes; promotes the training of staff; and fosters the development of professional attitudes and behavior. Many evaluations have revealed ambiguous outcomes, leaving administrators, planners, and providers with essentially no explanation as to *why*. This has led to interest in issues of program input and the process by which the program is put into place. This addresses the issue of *how* the program is to work. There is also a growing awareness of the importance of theory in program operation. This addresses the issue of *why* the program is intended to have certain effects. The need for assessing program impact remains, that is, the question of whether and to what extent the program has an effect. But the answer to this question becomes less useful without answers to *how* and *why* the program operates as it does.

A number of developments have been identified that will require greater attention and sophistication of health services administrators, providers, and others entrusted with determining public policy in the health arena. Among these were (1) the growing involvement of the federal government in health services financing and provision, (2) continued growth of new technology, (3) growing demands for public accountability, and (4) large-scale programmatic interventions. These factors are themselves interrelated, creating an ever more complex environment for the evaluation of health care programs. These forces will continue to give rise to the questions of *how, why,* and *to what extent*. These questions are at the center of both administrative rationality and evaluative research and form the common link between the two. As such, program evaluations take on added significance for practicing administrators, planners, and providers.

Program evaluation is defined as the use of scientific method (or an approximation) in judging the worth of a particular program to provide information to decision-makers and policy-makers in a position to improve the program, extend it to other sites, or cut back or abolish the program so that resources may be allocated to other efforts. Program evaluations frequently serve as examples of policy research and as input into the policy analysis process. Program evaluation differs from nonevaluative research in that program evaluation is usually less directly concerned with advancing understanding of basic social phenomena.

The reasons for evaluating a specific program will differ depending on the interested parties. The perspectives of the agency, the program administrator, the funding agency, the public or client group, and the evaluator are likely to differ in varying degrees about (1) the objectives to be evaluated, (2) the types of evaluation to be conducted, (3) the research design to be employed, (4) the relevant measures of program input, process, and impact, (5) the collection of data, (6) the analysis of data, (7) the inferences to be drawn from the data, and (8) the uses to which the findings are to be put. Chapter 2 addresses the first two issues concerning program objectives and the type of evaluation to be employed. Chapter 3 focuses on issues of research design. Chapter 4 is concerned with measurement, data collection, and analysis issues. Chapter 5 deals explicitly with the political and administrative issues affecting both the conduct of program evaluations and the uses to which they are put. Chapter 6 is devoted to a discussion of major policy issues facing those involved in the evaluation of health care programs. (Some of these issues have been mentioned in this chapter.)

Glossary

health policy analysis Involves the compilation and evaluation of existing research, information, and informed judgment concerning the implications (pro and con) of alternative strategies for dealing with a specific problem or set of problems associated with the delivery of health services.

health policy research Investigations directed toward specific problems associated with the delivery of health services, the results of which are to be used, in the short or long run, by those in a position to make decisions regarding the problem or issue at hand.

impact evaluation (summative evaluation) The assessment of program outcomes, for example, measuring the effect of a hypertension patient-education program through age-adjusted blood pressure readings.

nonevaluative research Use of the scientific method, or an approximation, to advance knowledge and understanding of a variety of social and physical phenomena. The primary purpose is to contribute to the further development of disciplinary knowledge.

process evaluation (formative evaluation) The assessment of the degree to which a program is implemented, for example, measuring the number of hypertension patients actually attending the education program.

program evaluation Use of the scientific method, or approximations, in assessing the degree to which an organized set of activities has reached intended objectives. The primary purpose is to inform the decisions of program operators.

References

1. Kane, R. L., Hanson, R., and Deniston, O. L.: Program evaluation: is it worth it? In Kane, R. L., editor: The challenges of community medicine, New York, 1974, Springer Publishing Co., Inc.
2. Williamson, J.: Health accounting and outcome measures of quality of care. In The hospital's role in assessing the quality of medical care, Fifteenth Annual Symposium on Hospital Affairs, Center for Health Administration Studies, University of Chicago, May, 1973, pp. 22-28.
3. Suchman, E.: Evaluative research: principles and practice in public service and social action programs, New York, 1967, Russell Sage Foundation, pp. 13, 14, 16-18.
4. Gustafson, D., and others: Roles and training for future health systems engineers, Educ. Health Admin. 2:25-60, 1975.
5. Weiss, C. H.: Evaluation research, Englewood Cliffs, N.J., 1972, Prentice-Hall, Inc.
6. Williams, W.: Implementation analysis and assessment, Policy Anal. 1:531-566, 1975.
7. Pressman, J. L., and Wildavsky, A. B.: Implementation, Berkeley, 1973, University of California Press.
8. Henderson, M., and Meinert, C. L.: A plea for a discipline of health and medical evaluation, Int. J. Epidemiol. 4:11-23, 1975.
9. Bernstein, I. N., and Freeman, H. E.: Academic and entrepreneurial research, New York, 1975, Russell Sage Foundation, p. 39.
10. Bice, T., Eichorn, R. L., and Klein, D. A.: Evaluation of public health programs. In Guttentag, M., and Struening, E. L., editors: Handbook of evaluation research, vol. 2, Beverly Hills, Calif., 1975, Sage Publications, Inc., pp. 605-620.
11. Cooper, B. S., and others: Compendium of national health expenditures data, Washington, D.C., 1976, Social Security Administration, Department of Health, Education and Welfare.
12. Brook, R.: Conference on future directions in health care: the dimensions of medicine, New York, December 10-11, 1975, sponsored by the Rockefeller Foundation, Blue Cross Association, Health Policy Program of the University of California, San Francisco, pp. 42-43.
13. Banta, D. H., and Fox, R. C.: Rural strains of health care team in a poverty community, Soc. Sci. Med. 6:697-721, 1972.
14. Newhouse, J. P.: A design for a health insurance experiment, Inquiry 1:5-27, March 11, 1974.
15. Perrow, C.: Goals and power structures—a historical case study. In Freidson, E., editor: The hospital of modern society, New York, 1963, The Free Press.
16. American Council on Education: University education for administration in hospitals, Washington, D.C., 1954, The Council.
17. Personal communication, 1977.
18. Knutson, A. L.: Evaluation for what? In Schulberg, H. C., and others, editors: Program evaluation in the health fields, New York, 1969, Behavioral Publications, Inc., pp. 42-50.
19. McCullough, P.: Training for evaluators. In Zusman, J., and Wurster, C. R., editors: Program evaluation: alcohol, drug abuse and mental health services, Lexington, Mass., 1975, Lexington Books, p. 248.

Suggested readings

Bice, T., Eichhorn, R., and Klein, D.: Evaluation of public health programs. In Guttentag, M., and Struening, E. L., editors: Handbook of evaluation research, vol. 2, Beverly Hills, Calif., 1975, Sage Publications, Inc. pp. 605-620.
Henderson, M. M., and Meinert, C. L.: A plea for a discipline of health and medical evaluation, Int. J. Epidemiol. 4:11-23, 1975.
Myers, B. A.: Evaluation of health services in the federal government. In Yaffe, R., and Zalkind, D., editors: Evaluation in health services delivery, New York, 1973, Engineering Foundation, pp. 2-7.
Suchman, E. A.: Evaluative research: principles and practice in public service and social action programs, New York, 1967, Russell Sage Foundation, pp. 11-26.

CHAPTER 2

The evaluation process

In this chapter, the evaluation process is looked at from the following perspectives: the specification of objectives, the delineation of all the elements in the program evaluation process, and the identification of specific categories of evaluation.

Although this may oversimplify a complex topic, program evaluation can be subdivided into three basic stages: (1) the specification of program objectives (the program planning stage); (2) the organization of resources to carry out the program (the program implementation stage); and (3) the assessment of program performance (the program impact stage). Each activity takes place within the context of the value structure of the participants and the larger society. This process is shown in Fig. 2. The following section raises issues pertaining to the specification of program objectives.

Specification of objectives

It is often observed that the reason little is known from the evaluations of many health care programs is that the right questions are frequently not asked in the first place. There is no more important task for program administrators, providers of care, policy-makers, and evaluators than to specify in clear, precise, and measurable terms the program objectives to be accomplished. Weiss refers to this as "formulating the question"[1] and, as noted in Chapter 1, it is likely to differ for each group involved in the process. The evaluators' task, however, is to assist (without imposing their own preconceptions) the parties involved in arriving at a reasonable degree of consensus on program objectives and a concrete level of measurement to ensure enough common ground from which an evaluation may proceed.

While these conditions are generally necessary, a word of caution is in order. There are situations in which it does not make sense to specify an objective in measurable terms. In fact, it is important to avoid the tendency to choose objectives based solely on whether they are measurable, when in fact they may not be at all the most important objectives of the program. Thus, objectives should be selected independently of the extent to which they can be measured. After the objectives have been listed and accepted as reasonable by all parties, then the process of developing operational indicators can proceed. However, if individuals are not able to specify objectives or if a great deal of conflict exists regarding what the operational indicators should be, serious consideration should be given to omitting the evaluation since its cost may far outweigh the benefit of its information for decision-making.

The process of specifying program objectives is essentially a matter of

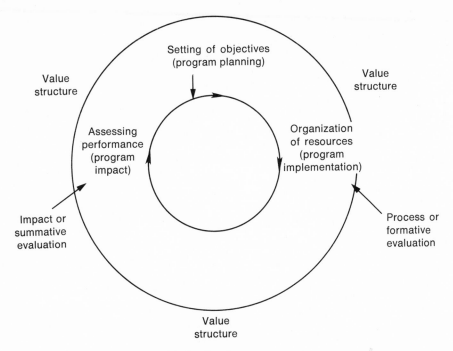

Fig. 2. Evaluation process.

answering the following question: "How will you know one when you see one?" This applies regardless of the issue at hand. It applies to assessing the impact of a physician continuing education program on quality of care, to assessing the effects of a transfer from hospital-based to community-based treatment for mental health patients, to assessing the effects of new health practitioners on patient compliance and costs of care, and to many other examples.

In brief, on what basis can one judge whether the program is, relatively speaking, a success or failure? How will one know?

Problems involved in specifying clear program objectives largely center around communication issues and the failure of the evaluator to ask specific and probing questions of those who want the program evaluated. This is illustrated in a rather humorous fashion by the following fable.

> Once upon a time in the land of Fuzz, King Aling called in his cousin Ding and commanded, "Go ye out into all of Fuzzland and find me the goodest of men, whom I shall reward for his goodness."
>
> "But how will I know one when I see one?" asked the Fuzzy.
>
> "Why, he will be *sincere*," scoffed the king, and whacked off a leg for his impertinence.
>
> So, the Fuzzy limped out to find a good man. But soon he returned, confused and empty-handed.
>
> "But how will I know one when I see one?" he asked again.

"Why, he will be *dedicated*," grumbled the king, and whacked off another leg for his impertinence.

So the Fuzzy hobbled away once more to look for the goodest of men. But again he returned, confused and empty-handed.

"But how will I know one when I see one?" he pleaded.

"Why, he will have *internalized his growing awareness*," fumed the king, and whacked off another leg for his impertinence.

So the Fuzzy, now on his last leg, hopped out to continue his search. In time, he returned with the wisest, most sincere, and dedicated Fuzzy in all of Fuzz-land, and stood him before the king.

"Why, this man won't do at all," roared the king. "He is much too thin to suit me." Whereupon he whacked off the last leg of the Fuzzy, who fell to the floor with a squishy thump.

The moral of this fable is that . . . *if you can't tell one when you see one, you may wind up without a leg to stand on.*[2]

To avoid fuzzy terminology, one must be able to (1) separate program abstractions from those describing program performance and (2) describe performances that represent the meaning of the program's objectives, that is, describe *specific outcomes* that, if achieved, will enable one to agree that the objective is also achieved. For example, if the objective of a program to introduce new health practitioners into an ambulatory clinic is to increase patients' access to care, will this objective have been accomplished if (1) the average patient waiting time is reduced by X percent, or (2) the length of time between making an appointment and the actual visit is reduced by X percent, or (3) X percent of patients report X units of greater satisfaction with access to care, or (4) various combinations of the above are brought about? Furthermore, on what basis does one set the level of improvement: 10 percent, 25 percent, 50 percent? In summary, useful objectives require (1) a statement of the specific behaviors or accomplishments to be examined and (2) specification of the "success" criteria for these behaviors.

A number of important dimensions of program objectives need to be identified, including the following:

1. *Nature or content of the objective*—is the program intended to produce changes in information, opinions, attitudes, or behavior? For example, some programs are primarily designed to change people's behavior (such as behavior modification programs for smokers) while others are designed to change attitudes (such as educational campaigns on the benefits of fluoridation).

2. *Ordering of objectives*—the level of abstraction at which the objective is stated. At *each* level of abstraction the objective should be *clearly* stated with a corresponding operational indicator which would permit one to say that the objective has been met. This will be elaborated on later.

3. *Target group*—for what specific group is the program intended? What are the geographic boundaries of the group? For example, is an ambulatory care clinic's outreach program designed to reach specific age, sex, ethnic categories? Is it aimed at a particular geographic area?

4. *Short-term versus long-term effects*—how quickly is the program intended to produce effects? For example, the development of a vaccine for polio can produce quite immediate effects, while the development of new manpower programs, such as the National Health Service Corps, or programs requiring new organizations (for example, Professional Standards Review) usually require at least several years before effects can be observed. In general, the more complex the program being initiated, the more diverse the target group to receive the program, and the more complex the environment in which the program must operate, the longer the time needed to observe program effects. It is with these programs that implementation assessments, or formative evaluations, become so important.

5. *Magnitude of effect*—how large an effect is expected? For example, is a fluoridation program intended to result in a 30 percent decrease in tooth decay, a 50 percent decrease, or a 75 percent decrease? Or will *any* decrease, no matter how small, be accepted as a positive indicator of program success?

6. *Stability of effect*—how long are the effects produced by the program intended to last? For many programs, the effects are meant to be permanent, but for others, particularly continuing education programs and programs involving changes in one's behavior, it is recognized that additional retraining or reexposure to the program is necessary.

7. *Multiplicity of objectives*—most programs have more than a single objective. These objectives may be conflicting. For example, an outreach program may increase access to care but may also increase program costs.

8. *Interrelatedness of objectives*—the objectives may be highly related and similar to each other or unrelated and dissimilar. An example of similar and related objectives is a program designed to increase patients' knowledge of hypertension and increase adherence with medical regimen. An example of a program with less similar and less related objectives is an outreach program in a poverty community designed to increase use of health services while at the same time intervene in the "cycle of poverty" within the community.

9. *Importance*—objectives will differ in importance. As noted earlier, individuals will often disagree on the importance of each objective. For example, in the case of university-based programs for the mentally retarded and developmentally disabled, faculty members are more likely to place greater importance on education and training, while direct care providers and community groups are more likely to emphasize service to clients.

10. *Unintended and unanticipated "second order" consequences*—the program may produce effects not intended but anticipated, or even unanticipated, by its initiators. For example, an unintended effect of a methadone maintenance program may be the further addiction (to methadone) of those who were not true addicts previously. It is important for those involved in the evaluation to try to think through in ad-

vance the various possible "side effects" of the program under question. This will be elaborated on in the following paragraphs.

Of the above characteristics, the following three deserve particular consideration: (1) the ordering of objectives, (2) the multiplicity of objectives, and (3) the unintended and/or unanticipated consequences of the objectives. Each will be discussed in turn.

Ordering of objectives

Program objectives, as Suchman notes, may be ordered from immediate to ultimate or, in current terminology, from lower order to higher order objectives.[3] Such ordering of objectives is important because it helps to forge the link between program design and implementation and the assessment of program impact. For example, lower order objectives are usually more concerned with *implementation*. They involve what Weiss calls input variables and "program operation" variables.[1] Examples of input variables include the human and capital resources available for program implementation (staffing patterns, facilities and equipment, financing, and so on); examples of program operation variables include issues of who is to do what, where, when, and how. These variables often comprise the *independent* variables in research investigation. Analysis of these variables and processes, as previously noted, is frequently termed *formative evaluation*. In contrast, as one moves toward ultimate or higher order objectives, the focus is centered on program *outcomes* or *impacts*. These often comprise the *dependent* variables in investigations. The concern is with determining *how much* of an effect the program produced. As previously indicated, this is frequently termed *summative evaluation*.

It is important to note that the ordering of objectives from immediate to ultimate (lower order to higher order) is a continuum and that certain *intermediate* level objectives serve as a link between the two. These objectives frequently involve the specification of particular subcomponents of the program involving what Weiss calls, "bridging variables."[1] In research terms, they may also be called *intervening* variables. For example, in analyzing the effectiveness of new health practitioners, one assumes that the knowledge and skills they have obtained through training can be implemented on the job and will result in beneficial outcomes. The "bridging variable" in this case becomes the particular combination of knowledge and skills that has been learned. Other such variables might include the organization of the practice and the attitudes and motivations of the new health practitioners themselves.

Intermediate level objectives involving bridging variables are intimately involved with the theory underlying the program's operation. For example, *why* is it that training nonphysician health providers may result in better (or equal) patient care at less cost? The theory is constructed along the following lines: (1) for a great many illnesses only a basic understanding of biology, anatomy, and physiology, together with certain technical skills, are needed to make a diagnosis and render treatment; (2) such knowledge and skills can be taught within a time period much shorter than that of medical school; (3) this training and knowledge can be introduced into current practice settings, and existing providers and patients will accept such practitioners; and (4) all this in turn will result in beneficial outcomes for the patient (better access, less cost, better quality). Thus, while program operation variables involving immediate objectives address the issue of *how* the program is to operate, the bridging variables involving intermediate level objectives address the issue of *why* the program is to produce certain intended effects.

In this light, it is important to realize that program failure may result from either a misspecification or an underdevelopment of theory (even though the program was successfully implemented), or from problems involved in getting the program "off the ground" (even though the program is theoretically sound), or from both. The misspecification of theory will force program planners, administrators, providers, and evaluators to rethink the major assumptions on which the program is based and to design alternative pathways to the goal. Problems of implementation will provide information on the conditions necessary for program success and the importance of building these conditions into the design of future programs.

This becomes clearer in the context of an example. Suppose there is interest in developing a program to improve the quality of care in hospitals. One begins by specifying and ordering the various objectives of this program, as shown in Fig. 3. The objectives are ordered from lower to higher, from immediate to ultimate, with the associated program operation, bridging, and im-

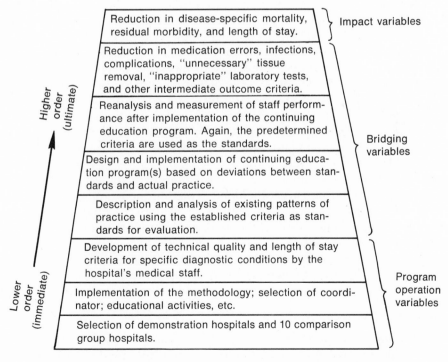

Fig. 3. Quality assurance program objectives: immediate to ultimate.

pact variables. The lower order objectives concerned with program operation variables involve selecting hospitals for the program, deciding how the program is to be introduced, selecting a coordinator, developing criteria, and so on. The intermediate order objectives involving the bridging variables and the underlying theory of the program include a description and analysis of current patterns of practice based on established criteria; the design and implementation of continuing education programs based on deviations between standards and actual practice; reanalysis of staff performance and examination of their relationship to such intermediate outcomes as medication errors, complication rates, and normal tissue removal. Finally, possible ultimate objectives of the program involving such impact variables as reduction in disease-specific mortality, morbidity, and length of stay are mentioned. In brief, by providing resources to develop and implement specific criteria of care, one assumes that it will be possible to judge performance against those criteria, to develop continuing education programs as needed, and to reevaluate performance and that this, in turn, will result in fewer "errors of treatment" and thus lead to better patient outcomes.

Specifying and ordering objectives force all parties to think through what the program is intended to do, why it is likely to be able to do it, and how it might be done. An *operational indicator* should also be associated with each level of objective. For example, in hospital selection, the indicator might be the percentage of hospitals that agreed to participate. In coordinator selection, relevant indicators might be the length of time it took each hospital to select a coordinator or the qualifications of the individual. In the case of quality of care criteria, relevant indicators might include the number of diseases for which criteria were developed or the acceptance of the criteria by the medical staff. Similar indicators can be developed for the remaining criteria. If the program fails to reduce disease-specific mortality or mobidity or complication rates, specific information is available for explanation. For example, the hospital may have waited too long to appoint a full-time coordinator, or perhaps the medical staff did not accept the established criteria, or perhaps the problem was not one of inadequate knowledge to be solved by continuing education programs but one of inadequate resources or resistance to change.

It should be obvious from the above that a program can be evaluated at *any* level of objective, but for any particular level chosen, the objectives preceding it in the hierarchy must also be included. Thus, in the example given, some may choose to conduct an implementation assessment (involving the first five or six objectives or some subset of them) on the grounds that it might take several years before the effects can be analyzed. Others may choose to incorporate immediately an analysis of the impact effects. This decision basically depends on the level of knowledge concerning the program and its likely effects.

Multiplicity of objectives

In addition to the multiplicity of objectives generated by the process of ordering objectives from immediate to ultimate, multiple objectives frequently exist for *each level* of the process. This is particularly true for intermediate and ultimate objectives. In the example of the quality assurance program, some individuals may have thought the primary intermediate objective was to develop hospital-based continuing education programs for medical staff, while others may have thought such education was the responsibility of the medical societies or various specialty associations. In regard to more outcome-oriented objectives, some observers may think that a primary objective is to contain costs by reducing unnecessary laboratory tests and other ancillary procedures, while others may think the primary objective is to rule out all reasonable alternative diagnoses regardless of increased numbers of laboratory tests or increased costs.

In addition to potential incompatibility among the program objectives, these objectives (even if internally compatible) may be incompatible with the goals and objectives of other programs and organization-wide goals and objectives. The program being evaluated does not exist in a vacuum, and those who are evaluating a given program must take into account the relationship of that program to other organization activities. The greater the extent to which the program being evaluated is interdependent with other organization programs, the greater the extent to which attention must be paid to multiple objectives, potentially incompatible objectives, and the process of program implementation itself. For example, the introduction of the primary care nursing concept into a hospital is likely to require more careful attention to implementation and specification of objectives than would the evaluation of a 4-day workweek in the hospital laundry. Hospital nursing units are highly interdependent with other hospital groups and activities (such as medical staff, admitting, laboratory, radiology), while the laundry department is more self-contained.

Where multiple program objectives exist, it is necessary to get the primary individuals involved to agree on a relative rank-ordering of the importance of each objective. Second, it is necessary to try to specify which particular set of program resources (inputs) and which particular subcomponents of the program are relevant for each objective. For example, if the purpose of a quality review program is to both contain costs and maintain or improve quality, then resources and activities involving preadmission screening would be relevant to the objective of containing costs, while the activities and resources devoted to auditing medical records would be relevant to the objective of maintaining quality but not to containing costs.

Unintended/unanticipated consequences

Again, to the extent the program is interdependent with other organizational activities and programs, it will produce unintended and unanticipated consequences. The goal of those involved in the evaluation is to *anticipate* such consequences, even though they are unintended. The issue is illustrated by the following example concerning installation of a fetal heart monitor in a community hospital.

> There is in the medical community the rather widespread assumption that any type of information that can be given to a physician is likely to improve the quality of care which that physician is capable of delivering. Consequently,

whenever a new device or piece of apparatus is developed which offers to provide extra information, there is almost an immediate market for it. It is not necessarily the case, however, that all information regardless of how correct it is will be utilized in a way that will inevitably increase the quality of care measures. In a community known to the writers, a local hospital acquired a fetal heart beat monitor in order to give the obstetrician improved and continuing information on the condition of the fetus while still inside the mother's body, presumably so that better planning for the care of the mother and the fetus and the birth process could be managed. When the fetal heart rate monitor was acquired by the hospital, the obstetricians adopted it and used it with considerable enthusiasm for it did give them more information about the progress of the fetus.

However, the important question is what the physicians do with the information once they have it. In this particular case, it appears that caesarian deliveries increased drastically since the acquisition of the fetal heart rate monitor. Whether the increase in caesarians represents the best judgment of the obstetrician for delivering a high quality infant or whether it represents a defensive practice of medicine, the fact of the matter is that any increase in caesarian deliveries is to be regarded as serious. The evaluation question arises around the issue of whether the quality of birth is actually improved by the caesarian section. Presumably, before the advent of the fetal heart rate monitor these babies were being born anyway, and since the rate of stillbirth in the hospital in question was always quite low, the important issue is whether the monitor improved infant health at and after birth rather than whether or not they survived the birth process.

In this case we do not know the actual value of the monitor for the birth process since no evaluation of the impact of this instrument has been done. It should also be recognized that the caesarian operation itself is not without wider impact upon these mothers since ordinarily they are encouraged to limit their subsequent family severely, thereby infringing upon their rights and interests in having children. It is also clear that, if the rates of caesarians get high enough, it might have implications for population growth. These broad questions should be studied along with the more immediate utilities of the heart monitor.

This case illustrates the need for a broad-based evaluation of the development of technology in medical care and the need to assess its impact on actual medical practices and subsequent health. Even though technology may improve some aspects of health, it is not necessarily true that the overall result will be positive.[4]

Various strategies exist for trying to anticipate such consequences. These include (1) becoming thoroughly familiar with the organization in which the program exists, (2) paying particular attention to those departments and programs that supply information or resources to the program under evaluation or that depend on it, (3) talking with intended clients or recipients of the program, (4) talking with people who honestly believe the program will fail, (5) communicating with kindred organizations, (6) contacting agencies which may have launched similar programs, (7) brainstorming, and (8) contacting other program evaluators to get their thoughts and suggestions.

Numerous possibilities exist for becoming familiar with the organization in which the program exists. These include reviewing organizational charts, policy documents, minutes of meetings, audit reports, and public media notices. Informal discussions can be held with people in positions at various levels of the organization. It may be useful, for example, to talk with people directly below and directly above the individual whose program is being evaluated. Their expectations of the program may be quite different from those of the people responsible for it.

Gathering input from those departments that supply information or other resources to the program or that depend on the program enables the evaluator to obtain a better understanding of operational constraints. This is particularly true when the activities of the program being evaluated are highly interdependent with other programs or departmental activities.

Communicating with intended clients, critics, kindred organizations, and organizations with similar programs can help to expand the universe of possible program outcomes. Brainstorming with individuals both inside and outside the organization can be useful. Nominal group[5] and Delphi[6] techniques for soliciting judgments can be used. Contacting other program evaluators experienced in evaluating similar programs can uncover additional unexpected and unanticipated consequences.

Finally, it may also be useful to ask oneself, "What is the worst possible thing that could go wrong with this program?" Having done all this, the evaluation is still likely to miss several unintended consequences. But the potential scope of program consequences will have been broadened and can be related back to intended objectives and to the plan for program implementation.

It should be noted that in employing these strategies, the evaluator adopts *neither* the perspective of assessing only attainment of goals nor of assessing only the system characteristics of the organization pursuing those goals.[7] Rather, the evaluator uses a combination of the two. The goal attainment model maintains that one must evaluate exclusively the objectives set by program participants, often those of the program administrator. It also assumes that objectives can be assessed separately, one at a time, and thus ignores the interrelatedness of program objectives. In contrast, the systems model is concerned with the entire organizational unit (or the entire organization itself) involved in the attainment of the objective. It focuses on the coordination, maintenance, and adaptation strategies of the group, and on balancing these processes with the attainment of objectives. The drawback to this approach is that the evaluator may become very involved in organizational processes beyond those necessary for the evaluation at hand. For example, to evaluate the clinical effectiveness of introducing nurse practitioners into a neighborhood health center, one need not know the details of the center's cash-flow status.

What is needed is a balance between goal attainment and systems perspectives. The evaluator needs to keep an eye on the specific program objective and at the same time have a basic understanding of the social context of the program. It keeps the evaluation team alert to serendipitous events which, although likely to result in negative consequences, may occasionally result in positive spin-offs as well.

Strategies for specifying objectives

One can identify a number of reasons why program administrators do not set objectives in precise terms. The most obvious reason is that, in the case of complex programs, this may be very difficult. In addition to recognizing inherent difficulty, program administrators do not wish to constrain their flexibility. Specification of objectives commits the program to a certain degree of visibility and communicates *intentions* to other parties. The program administrator may worry that too much is expected from the program. This is particularly true with a government-financed program in which the reality of program operation may not live up to legislative rhetoric and public media expectations.[8]

Given such constraints, four techniques are particularly helpful for writing useful objectives: (1) using strong verbs, (2) stating only one purpose or aim, (3) specifying a single end-product or result, and (4) specifying the expected time for achievement.[9]

A *"strong" verb is an action-oriented verb* which describes an observable or measurable behavior that will occur. For example, "to *increase* the use of health education materials" is an action-oriented statement involving behavior that can be observed. In contrast, "to *promote* greater use of health education materials" is a weaker and less specific statement. The term "promote" is subject to many interpretations. Examples of action-oriented, strong verbs include: "to write," "to meet," "to find," "to increase," "to sign." Examples of weaker, nonspecific verbs include: "to understand," "to encourage," "to enhance," "to promote."

A second useful suggestion for writing a clear objective is to *state only a single aim or purpose.* Most programs will, of course, have multiple objectives but *within each* objective only a single purpose should be delineated. An objective that states two or more purposes or desired outcomes may well require different implementation and assessment strategies, making achievement of the objective difficult to determine. For example, the statement "to begin three prenatal classes for pregnant women and provide outreach transportation services to accommodate twenty-five women per class" create difficulties. This objective contains two aims—to provide prenatal classes *and* to provide outreach services. If one aim is accomplished but not the other, to what extent has the objective been met? It is better to state a single aim for each objective, such as, *"start three prenatal classes for pregnant women," "provide outreach services to twenty-five pregnant women per class."*

Specifying a single end-product or result is a third technique contributing to a useful objective. For example, the statement "to begin *three* prenatal classes for pregnant women by *subcontracting* with City Memorial Hospital" contains two results, namely, the three classes and the subcontract. It is better to state these objectives separately, particularly since one is a higher order objective (to begin three prenatal classes) which depends partly on fulfillment of a lower order objective (to establish a subcontract).

A clearly written objective must have *both* a single aim and a single end-product or result. For example, the statement "to establish communication with the Health Systems Agency" indicates the aim but not the desired end-product or result. What constitutes evidence of communication—telephone calls, meetings, reports? Failure to specify a clear end-product makes it extremely difficult for assessment to take place.

The reverse is equally true. That is, statements can exist that specify an end-product but no aim or purpose. "To provide all monthly discharge abstracts to the Commission on Professional and Hospital Activities" is an example of a statement with an end-product but no aim or purpose. The implicit aim may be to improve medical staff accountability and management or to improve the quality of medical care, but it is not clear that submitting case abstracts will meet this objective, nor can the objective be assessed in a meaningful way without such a statement of purpose. Those involved in writing and evaluating objectives need to keep two questions in mind. First, would anyone reading the objective, with or without knowledge of the program, find the *same purpose* as the one intended? Second, what visible, measurable, or tangible results are present as evidence that the objective has been met? Purpose or aim describes what will be done; end-product or result describes evidence that will exist when it has been done. This is assurance that you "know one when you see one."

Finally, it is useful to specify the time of *expected achievement* of the objective. The statement "to establish a walk-in clinic as soon as possible" is not a useful objective because of the vagueness of "as soon as possible." It is far more useful to specify a target date or, in cases where considerable doubt exists, a range of target dates; for example, "sometime between March 1 and March 30."

Each of these suggestions is relatively simple and straightforward. Yet even casual examination of most health services program objectives will indicate shortcomings in one or more of these areas. It is often the simple and obvious points that are most ignored; yet, at the same time, they represent some of the most useful ingredients in implementing a program and assessing its results.

While these represent specific techniques that can be useful in writing clearer objectives, Weiss has summarized some general strategies evaluators can use to aid people in specifying objectives.[1] These include (1) outlining the relevant questions and permitting program people to arrive at a consensus, (2) collecting as much information as possible about the program and letting the evaluator actually formulate the objectives, (3) encouraging collaboration between the evaluator and the program people so that both formulate possible objectives and then agree to a manageable and realistic set, and (4) avoiding specific statements of objectives and, instead, settling for a more open-ended exploratory study. Of the four strategies, the second (letting the evaluator formulate the objectives) is the most dangerous because the program participants can readily dismiss the results of the evaluation by saying that "it wasn't really what they had in mind at all." The third approach, mutual collaboration, probably offers the greatest advantage since the evaluator is able to suggest to program personnel how their objectives might be sharpened, while at the same time letting program personnel make the final determination of objectives. Various small group process strategies, such as the nominal group[5] or Delphi[6] techniques cited earlier, can be used to assist program personnel in arriving at specifically stated objectives. In all these approaches, however, the objectives may change in midstream. Therefore, evaluators need to keep in contact with program personnel and operations.

Of particular importance to the evaluator in specifying objectives is to recognize that most programs take place within organizations. Thus, the role of the specific program must be viewed within the context of the overall system-wide goals of the organization. For example, the primary objective of a family medical care program in a university teaching hospital may be to provide accessible and continuous care to people living in its immediate area. From the hospital's viewpoint, however, the main objective may be to provide a source of patient referral for teaching and research purposes. To evaluate such a program only for its impact on accessibility and continuity of care misses half the picture. Furthermore, without knowledge of the larger institutional objectives it becomes more difficult to understand why the program may not achieve these objectives.

In summary, attention must be paid to both program objectives and the relationship of these objectives to larger organizational objectives. There is no need to debate further the systems versus goal models of evaluation. Both perspectives need to be recognized. What determines the relative degree of emphasis is the extent to which the program to be evaluated is tightly connected with other parts of the organization. If it is tightly connected, greater attention needs to be paid to system goals.

While most programs exist within organizations, it is sometimes the case that *organizations are created* for the purpose of administering a given program. The Professional Standards Review Organizations (PSROs) operating in various states are prime examples. In such cases, the evaluator needs to pay particular attention to how the organization established itself as a viable entity and how this, in turn, may affect the particular program being implemented. For example, in the case of PSROs the political relationships of the designated bodies with other regulatory bodies (such as health systems agencies or hospital rate review commissions) and the attitudes of provider groups (for example, state hospital associations) will affect the implementation of quality assurance programs.

The end-result of the objective-setting process should usually be the development of action-oriented statements with associated operational indicators. Three examples are provided below.

Objective	*Operational indicator*
1. Provide information on hypertension treatment to improve physicians' knowledge of treatment of hypertension.	1. A 25 percent improvement in post-test versus pretest examination scores.
2. Increase the percentage of recommended physician practices in the treatment of hypertension.	2. A 30 percent increase in the percentage of recommended physician practices performed from postprogram versus preprogram.
3. Lower the age-adjusted blood pressure of patients with hypertension.	3. Ninety percent of all treated patients should have blood pressures within age-adjusted normal levels within 12 months.

Two observations may be made regarding these examples. The first is the use of verbs in the statement of objectives ("provide," "improve," "lower"). A general guideline is that the higher the ratio of verbs to nouns in the statement of objectives, the greater the likelihood that the objective will be subject to evaluation.

The second observation concerns the delineation of operational indicators. Program personnel often find this more difficult than stating objectives. Attaching numbers to statements somehow intensifies the burden of program responsibility. As previously suggested, administrators frequently deal with problems in which a sign of *good management* is to be more general than specific in one's objectives in order to allow for needed flexibility and to control information one does not wish to share with others. Thus, the tendency is to be the opposite of operationally specific. Several strategies can be used by evaluators to assist program personnel in overcoming this resistance. First, it is not necessary to develop point estimates. Ranges of program impact such as a 15 to 30 percent improvement in some scores may be sufficient to make an evaluation of program success. Second, it is often useful for the evaluator to meet with program personnel and review past performance on baseline data in the light of available resources and the difficulty of the problem being addressed. This process may assist program personnel in setting realistic indicators. Third, the situation might be structured in such a way that the administrator would be held responsible only for failure to perform certain activities associated with implementing the program. The administrator would not be held responsible for failure in the underlying theory of the program or for inherent difficulties in implementation not associated with the administrator's own responsibilities. To the extent possible, an indicator or a set of indicators should be determined by which all concerned will agree that if these indicators are attained the program will be considered a success.

Delineation of program elements

Once the program's objectives have been specified and operational indicators determined, they can be placed in context with all the elements of the program. A major weakness of most evaluation research, particularly in the health field, is that the exact nature of the program intervention or "treatment" is never clearly specified. Sometimes the boundaries of the program as well as specific subcomponents are ill-defined. This is particularly true if the program is an outgrowth of a preexisting program, represents an addition to a current program, or is tightly connected with other programs and activities in the organization. In such situations it is often difficult to know exactly what the program was, and therefore difficult to attribute success or failure to the program itself. This is particularly true if the program is somewhat abstruse in character. For example, it is generally more difficult to assess mental health programs than immunization programs.

Even when these circumstances do not hold, the difficulty of determining the nature of the program intervention frequently remains, because of the complexity of the programs, particularly such large-scale social interventions as the Rand Health Insurance Experiment or the Robert Wood Johnson

Foundation's program to establish hospital-sponsored primary care group practices. It can also be true of smaller efforts aimed at introducing a new program into a single organization. For example, a health maintenance organization's decision to introduce nurse practitioners raises a number of programmatic issues, such as the personalities of the individuals being employed, specification of their duties, and delineation of relationships with other providers, to name but a few.

Despite such obstacles, attempts must be made to specify as clearly as possible, in advance, all the elements of a particular program intervention. Failure to do so not only clouds the inferences that can be drawn from program results but also diminishes the value of the information which can be used for decision-making. The question of *how* the program operated to produce the result cannot be addressed. The learning feedback loop to corrective action is truncated. The administrator or provider has no idea which specific elements of the program contributed to the end-result and which were unrelated.

A useful way of delineating program elements is to develop a *model*. Here, the evaluator lays out in sequential fashion the major elements of the program and situation to be analyzed. This approach combines and adapts the views of Suchman[3] and Weiss[1] and consists of five features: (1) preexisting conditions, (2) program components, (3) intervening events, (4) impact, and (5) consequences. The general model is shown in Table 1 and is described next.

Preexisting conditions

In order to understand the specific characteristics of a new program, one must know something about the existing state of the target group and the organization and various factors in the environment of both. It is necessary to

Table 1. Model for delineating program elements in the evaluation process

Preexisting conditions	Program components	Intervening events	Impact	Consequences
The current state of the target group to be affected The organization implementing the program The degree of interdependence with other programs The larger environment in which both the target group and the organization function	Inputs 1. Program objectives 2. Resources Activities	Factors which will affect how the program operates during the course of the evaluation; these factors may be either internal or external to the organization	Extent to which operational indicators of objectives are attained	Effects of attaining the objective

separate figure from field. Among the characteristics of the target group to consider are sociodemographic information and current measures on the variables which the program is intended to change (such as access to medical care, continuity of care, health status). Information on the organization would include its current structure, services, philosophy, and resources.

Particularly important is the need to determine the degree to which the program is interdependent with other programs and activities of the organization. Thompson discusses three types of interdependence relevant to program evaluation.[10] These are pooled, sequential, and reciprocal interdependence. Pooled interdependence exists when the programs or activities have no direct relationship or exchanges with each other but, rather, their outputs must be coordinated at some higher level in the organization. Sequential interdependence exists when program A depends on resources of program B, or program B needs to complete an activity before program A can operate. Reciprocal interdependence exists when both programs are mutually dependent on each other for resources and/or activities. As a general observation, the extent to which the program is reciprocally interdependent with others determines how difficult it will be to delineate program elements and assess program effects.

Finally, information on the environment would include data related to the geographic, political, and economic factors affecting both the target group and the organization delivering the program.

Program components

Program components comprise both inputs and activities. The inputs of particular programs to be evaluated would include program objectives, financial and personnel resources, staffing patterns, location of the program, length of time, size, and sponsorship. Other inputs might include the motivations and perceptions of the program participants as opposed to their sociodemographic characteristics, which are considered preexisting conditions. Relevant motivational and perceptual variables might include personal aspirations and expectations, family attitudes, and degree of support available from friends and family. Although it is useful to make an exhaustive list of inputs to ensure that nothing has been overlooked, it is usually necessary to focus on only a few. In such cases, a useful decision-rule is to select those inputs that are most likely to be under the program's control, such as staffing patterns or hours of service.

Program activities refer to particular actions carried out in support of program objectives by the use of other program inputs. Weiss' notion of *program operation* variables and *bridging* variables is again relevant.[1] The program operation variables refer specifically to implementation activities. Who is doing what to whom, with what resources, and within what period of time? The bridging variables refer to the overall sequence of events involved in going from the program inputs to the achievement of program outcomes. For example, in a program designed to increase utilization of physician services, intervening processes reflecting bridging variables might include removal of financial barriers (drawing on economic theory) and patient and provider education (drawing on learning theories).

A useful approach to delineating program activities would be to develop two sets of flow charts. The first would outline the major activities of each individual associated with the program and would primarily include program operation variables. The second would link the activities of all the relevant parties and would primarily involve bridging variables. Separate flow charts should be developed for each major program objective since it is unlikely that the same set of activities or sequence of events will contribute equally to all objectives.

Intervening events

The delineation of program inputs and activities and their separation from preexisting conditions represent major factors in specifying the nature of the program to be evaluated. An additional factor is the specification of key intervening events. These refer to activities going on within the organization itself, or among target group participants, or in the larger environment which may affect and interact with the program itself. Examples include merger of the organization with another organization, changes in the types of clients receiving program services, unexpected changes in program leadership, and major changes in the larger political economy (for example, introduction of national health insurance). Such factors may alter the nature of program inputs and activities. As will be seen in Chapter 3, these factors can sometimes be controlled through the appropriate choice of evaluation design. However, since the "most appropriate" designs are often difficult to implement in practice, it is important to try to specify such factors in advance so that they can be carefully studied for possible impact on program outcomes, in the absence of evaluation designs that might automatically rule them out as competing explanations for any effects that may be observed.

Impacts and consequences

The final two elements of the process model refer to the program's actual impact and associated consequences. If multiple objectives have been set, it is important to link other program inputs and activities and possible intervening events to each objective. As indicated earlier, it should be possible to assess each objective according to the extent to which the operational indicator has been met. Finally, to complete the model, it is useful to list various consequences (to both the recipients and the organization) of the program's impact. For example, the consequences of a successful child immunization program may be healthier children, fewer school absence days, and perhaps a more positive attitude toward health care practices. For the organization, consequences may include higher employee morale and renewed federal funding.

The model has been described in fairly general terms. Table 2 offers a concrete illustration using as an example a program designed to improve the quality of medical care in hospitals. By going through such an exercise, the evaluator is better able to pinpoint the *reasons why* the program did or did not have the intended effect, or did not have as great an impact as intended, or resulted in unintended consequences. For example, a hospital's apparent failure to lower its mortality rate may not be due to the failure of the complete

Table 2. Model for evaluating a quality assurance program

Preexisting conditions	Program components	Intervening events	Impact	Consequences

Hospital characteristics
1. Bed size
2. Patient mix
3. Staffing patterns
Medical staff organization
1. Percent primary care (family practice, internal medicine, pediatrics, obstetrics-gynecology)
2. Percent specialty
3. Departmental structure
4. Committee structure
5. Bylaws
6. Credential process, etc.
Previous audit activities
Medical staff attitudes toward quality assurance program
Hospital-wide attitudes toward quality assurance program
Relationship to nurse audit activities, utilization review programs, etc.
	Inputs
	1. Program objectives
	2. Resources
	  a. A half-time equivalent director of medical education
	  b. Program coordinator
	  c. Data abstracters
	  d. Data analysts
	  e. Office space
	  f. Supplies
	  g. Secretarial assistance
	Activities
	1. Hire or appoint individuals to the above positions
	2. Secure the backup support
	3. Decide what conditions are to be evaluated
	4. Decide sampling scheme for selection of conditions
	5. Develop criteria
	6. Make initial assessment
	7. Provide feedback of results
	8. Provide continuing education
	9. Reassess
		External
		1. PSRO activity
		2. Related continuing education programs
		Internal
		1. Medical staff reorganization
		2. Hospital reorganization
			Reduced disease-specific mortality
			Reduced disease-specific morbidity
				Greater patient satisfaction
				"Healthier" populations
				Increased medical staff pride
				Increased community respect for the hospital

quality assurance program but rather may be traced to a specific subcomponent, such as selection of conditions in which mortality rates are not a good outcome indicator of quality of care. Or, the program may have failed in its impact due to deficiencies in program implementation, for example, the inability to hire enough staff to ensure that the data is fed back to the medical staff in a timely and informative manner. This is the type of information which is most useful to the administrator, who has to have an answer to the question, "What is the next step?"

Categories of evaluation

It is possible to evaluate a program from several different perspectives. Suchman has summarized these in terms of (1) effort, (2) performance, (3) adequacy of performance, (4) efficiency, and (5) process.[3] The categories of evaluation are closely related to the objectives chosen for the program. *Effort* refers to the amount of energy which goes into a program. In terms of the quality assurance example, it refers to the number of manhours involved, the costs involved, the number of records reviewed, and so on. It is related to the lower order objectives shown in Fig. 3, p. 21. *Performance* asks what results were achieved with the given effort; that is, to what extent were mortality rates, postoperative complications, adverse drug reactions, and so on, reduced. It is related to the higher order objectives shown in Fig. 3. *Adequacy of performance* compares the level of performance achieved to the level of achievement realistically possible or to the level of need associated with the problem. For example, an initial evaluation of the quality assurance program may reveal a 20 percent decrease in postoperative complication rates, but the hospital's administrators and medical staff may know that another hospital of similar size and patient mix has a rate which is still lower by an additional 10 percentage points. Thus, they may believe that it is realistically possible to reduce their own rate further. Such information, coupled with data on costs, helps administrators to decide whether a program should be expanded.

Efficiency focuses on the issue of whether there is a less costly way of achieving the same results. For example, is it possible that a 20 percent reduction in postoperative complication rates could be achieved with less quality assurance program staff? Or could it be achieved by reviewing fewer conditions? External funding agencies are increasingly interested in issues of program efficiency. If two programs are about equally effective (achieve approximately the same results), the program which costs less has a greater probability of being re-funded. Specific cost-benefit and cost-effectiveness issues are discussed in Chapter 3. Finally, *process evaluation* focuses on the previously mentioned questions of how and why a program does or does not work. Again, the question of *how* addresses program implementation issues and primarily involves consideration of input variables and activities. The question of *why* is concerned with the underlying theory of program operation and is primarily concerned with bridging variables for the quality assurance evaluator. Implementation of quality assurance methodology and continuing education programs (see Fig. 3) represent objectives related to process evaluation categories.

Summary

This chapter has focused on the process of evaluation in terms of specification of program objectives, program elements, and evaluation categories. The importance of clearly specified objectives with associated operational indicators has been stressed. Techniques were suggested for writing clearer objectives and various strategies were presented for working with program personnel in developing such objectives. Special emphasis was given to the ordering of program objectives, the existence of multiple objectives, and the need to consider unintended consequences. Several suggestions for organizing program elements were also made. These involved a delineation of preexisting conditions, inputs and activities, intervening events, program impacts, and program consequences. Finally, five different categories of evaluation were discussed, including evaluation of effort, performance, adequacy of performance, efficiency, and process.

Together, Chapters 1 and 2 have provided a foundation for considering the evaluation design issues to be presented in Chapter 3.

Glossary

higher order objective The ultimate objective of the program. In research terms, the dependent variable to be assessed and explained; for example, to increase the health status of a defined group of people.

lower order objective Immediate or intermediate objectives, such as to have a full-time director of medical education or to conduct continuing education programs. It is important to note that higher order objectives generally depend on the completion of lower order objectives. It is also important to note that the determination of higher order and lower order objectives is *relative* to the nature of the program being assessed. For example, in some cases, the development of a continuing education program may be the ultimate higher order objective, with the inputs and processes leading up to this serving as the lower order intermediate objectives.

input variables Human and capital resources to be used by the program.

program operation variables Specification of who is to do what, where, when, and how.

independent variables Variables believed to affect program results. Independent variables primarily include input and program operation variables, as defined above.

bridging variables Also can be considered as *intervening* variables. They are concerned with subcomponents of a program and tend to link immediate and ultimate objectives. For example, if the ultimate objective (dependent variable) of a quality assurance program is to reduce diagnostic-specific complication rates, then a continuing education program might be viewed as a bridging or intervening variable through which the immediate objective (independent variable) of hiring a full-time director of medical education operates. In brief, one wants to assess the impact of a full-time director of medical education on diagnostic-specific complication rates but needs to recognize that certain bridging or intervening variables such as continuing education programs are likely to affect this outcome. Part of the effect of hiring a full-time director of medical education on complication rates may operate directly while part may operate indirectly through this person's development of various programs. Bridging variables are primarily concerned with *why* the program is intended to produce certain effects.

process model A diagram which sequentially lays out the major elements and factors affecting a program.

preexisting conditions Factors which exist before the program is put into place; for example, sociodemographic characteristics of the community to be served, organizational characteristics, and so on.

program components The inputs and activities which will comprise the operation of the program. Inputs include capital and labor, including the motivations, values, and perception of those involved with the program. Activities include specification of who is going to do what to whom with what resources and within what period of time.

intervening events Activities within the organization itself, the clients being served, or the larger environment which may affect how the program operates and its eventual results; examples include organizational mergers, change in leadership, and changes in the larger political economy within which the program operates.

intended impact The end-result change in behavior which the program is intended to affect; for example, an increase in the number of pregnant women receiving earlier prenatal examination.

consequences The effects (often long-term) of achieving the program's objectives; for example, in regard to the above-mentioned prenatal program, a hoped-for consequence would be an increase in the number of healthy children.

evaluation of effort Assessing the amount of energy which goes into the program: manhours, activities performed, and so on.

evaluation of performance Assessing the results achieved from the effort which went into the program.

evaluation of adequacy of performance Assessing levels of performance in comparison with the level of possible achievement or the level of need associated with the problem.

evaluation of efficiency Assessing whether the program results could have been achieved in a less costly manner.

evaluation of process Assessing how and why the program does or does not work.

Sample problem exercises

1. Imagine that you have just been appointed administrative director of a newly funded, hospital-based primary care group practice. The general purpose of the group practice is to improve the community's access to health services and relieve the current volume of patients visiting the hospital's emergency room.

You have been asked to develop a list of objectives for the group. This list will be discussed with the group's staff and hospital officials. It is intended that it will be used to evaluate the group's performance.

In developing the list of objectives, you should keep in mind the following questions:

    a. What general difference or change do you want to bring about in various groups of people—staff physicians, employees, patients, community groups, and so on?

    b. What specific behavior or accomplishments will you examine as indicators that the general difference or change is occurring?

2. Keeping in mind the criteria of strong, action-oriented verbs, single aims, single end-products, and specified time-periods, you are to evaluate the usefulness of the following three objectives:

    a. To meet the health care needs of patients by providing comprehensive and continuous care

    b. To reduce per-patient costs through the use of sound fiscal management and prudent, efficient use of available resources

    c. To have in operation within 1 year a partial service hospital which will provide health services to 5,000 rural residents

3. Assign the following reading to the class: Skipper, J. K., and Leonard, R. C.: Children, stress, and hospitalization: a field experiment, *J. Health Soc. Behav.* 9:275-287, 1968. Upon completion of this reading, the student is to diagram the process model describing the nature of the program under study. Elements of such a model should include the preexisting conditions, delineation of program components, possible intervening events, intended impacts, and possible consequences.

References

1. Weiss, C.: Evaluation research, Englewood Cliffs, N.J., 1972, Prentice-Hall, Inc., pp. 24, 28-29, 46-50.
2. Mager, R. F.: Goal analysis, Belmont, Calif., 1972, Fearon Publishers.
3. Suchman, E.: Evaluative research: principles and practice in public service and social action programs, New York, 1967, Russell Sage Foundation, pp. 60-68, 84.
4. D'Acosta, A., and Sechrest, L.: Program evaluation for health administrators, A.U.P.H.A. Task Force on Teaching of the Health and Behavioral Sciences, September, 1976, pp. 83-84.
5. Delbecq, A., VandeVen, A., and Gustafson, D.: Group techniques for program planning, Glenview, Ill., 1975, Scott, Foresman and Company.
6. Dalkey, N. C.: DELPHI, Santa Monica, Calif., 1967, The Rand Corporation.
7. Etzioni, A.: Two approaches to organizational analysis: a critique and a suggestion, Admin. Sci. Q. 5:257-278, 1960.
8. Mechanic, D.: The growth of bureaucratic medicine, New York, 1976, John Wiley & Sons, Inc., p. 187.
9. Kirschner Associates, Inc.: Programs for older Americans: objective setting and monitoring; a reference manual, Washington, D.C., 1975, Department of Health, Education and Welfare, Office of Human Development.
10. Thompson, J. D.: Organizations in action, New York, 1967, McGraw-Hill Book Co.

Suggested readings

Deutscher, I.: Toward avoiding the goal-trap in evaluation research, Paper presented at the American Sociological Association annual meeting, Montreal, Canada, August, 1974.

Kirschner Associates, Inc.: Programs for older Americans: objective setting and monitoring; a reference manual, Washington, D.C., 1975, Department of Health, Education and Welfare, Office of Human Development.

Mager, R. F.: Goal analysis, Belmont, Calif., 1972, Fearon Publishers.

Seeman, M., and Evans, J.: Output indicators and informal organization, Am. Sociol. Rev. 26:193-204, 1961; also in Lyden, F. J., editor: Policies, decisions, and organizations, New York, 1969, Appleton-Century-Crofts.

Sims, N. H.: Clinic self-evaluation manual for the determination and improvement of clinic efficiency, Washington, D.C., 1971, Department of Health, Education and Welfare, Maternal and Child Health Services.

Suchman, E. A.: Evaluative research: principles and practice in public service and social action programs, New York, 1967, Russell Sage Foundation, pp. 51-73.

Weiss, C.: Evaluation research: methods of assessing program effectiveness, Englewood Cliffs, N.J., 1972, Prentice-Hall, Inc., pp. 24-59.

CHAPTER 3 Evaluation designs

In this chapter, basic concepts and techniques for designing and executing program evaluations are discussed. Issues include (1) threats to validity, (2) pros and cons of different types of experimental and quasi-experimental designs, (3) randomization, (4) sampling, and (5) cost-benefit and cost-effectiveness analyses. Several examples are provided to illustrate major points, and an example of an evaluation design is presented in Appendix A. Issues concerning reliability and validity of measurement, data collection methods, and data analysis strategies are discussed in Chapter 4.

Future administrators, providers, and planners need to comprehend, apply, and evaluate the material presented in this chapter because of the significance of program evaluation to future roles. Mastery of the material contained in this chapter will not make the future administrator, provider, or planner an "expert" in evaluation research but will provide sufficient knowledge and skills to enable one to cooperate with experts in conducting evaluations. Furthermore, it will help future administrators, providers, and planners to recognize the complexity of the evaluation process without feeling overwhelmed, and will encourage a greater number of informed evaluations to be undertaken.

Validity of program results

The two major questions to be addressed in impact or outcome evaluations (summative evaluations) are (1) to what extent are the program effects really due to the program rather than competing explanations (the issue of causality), and (2) to what extent can results be generalized to other situations? The first issue concerns the internal validity of the evaluation results and the second concerns the external validity of the results. Internal validity is more important than external validity because, without first knowing whether the results can really be attributed to the program, one cannot generalize to other situations. The most common threats to internal and external validity are discussed here.

Threats to internal validity

Imagine yourself as the administrator of the outpatient clinics of a large urban hospital. One of your first assignments is to improve access to medical care, and you are told that a major problem appears to be the individual patient's lack of knowledge regarding health conditions in general and symptoms in particular. You are also told that a program designed to improve the individual's knowledge of common health conditions and symptoms was conducted during the past year. Anxious to get started, you run across a copy of the report of this program. In reviewing this report you find that the program consisted of five half-hour lecture-discussion sessions given once a week to a group of 100 outpatients. The participants' knowledge of common diseases and symptoms was not tested before introducing the program. Upon completion of the program, participants were given a questionnaire testing their knowledge of common diseases and symptoms. The type of design employed might be diagrammed as follows:

$$X \quad O$$
where X represents the program
and O the observation or measurement

Such a design is frequently called a *one-shot case study*.

Individuals conducting the study felt that the results were "encouraging" and that the program merited continued support. Having taken a course on program evaluation in graduate school, you have serious doubts as to the validity of this conclusion and outline the reasons for your doubt as follows.

History effects. First, the results could be due to a particular event or experience of the participants which occurred sometime between the beginning of the program and its termination. For example, articles in newspapers, or an educational television program devoted to health topics, or even the experience of receiving medical care itself during the study period could all serve as alternative explanations for the scores obtained, rather than the educational program itself. Such examples may be considered historical factors. *History*, in the sense of discrete events which occur between the beginning and end of a program, constitutes one general threat to validity.

Maturation effects. Second, the results could be due to systematic changes (mental or physical) going on within the program participants themselves. Examples might include increasing boredom with the program as it continued to evolve, or, in the case of patients with chronic diseases, a gradual increase in familiarity with and knowledge of the disease. Such efforts may be termed *maturation effects*, that is, events or processes occurring inside the individual as a function of time. They are a second general threat to validity and are to be distinguished from history in that maturation effects refer to events happening *inside* the individual while history refers to discrete events occurring *outside* the individual. Maturation is particularly likely to affect internal validity of program results the longer the time interval between the beginning of the study and the final measurement of results. For example, if one were attempting to assess the impact of a change in diet or blood cholesterol levels over a 2-year period, one might find that the cholesterol levels had actually increased. This does not necessarily mean that the diet change was a failure. Rather, the results might be due to the fact that the program participants aged 2 years over the course of the treatment.

Testing effects. A colleague suggests to you that the evaluation would have been more useful if there had been a testing of the participants' knowledge of disease *before* the program began. This can be diagrammed as

$$O_1 \; X \; O_2$$

and is commonly referred to as the *one group pretest-posttest design*. In this fashion, one could evaluate the degree of change (increase or decrease) in participants' knowledge before versus after receiving the educational program. But upon close inspection you realize that this adds little to the overall evaluation, and in fact creates several additional problems.

You recognize that the final knowledge scores may be due not to the effect of the program itself but to the fact that the test was taken *before*; that is, during the pretest phase of the program, the initial test may have communicated knowledge such that program participants would naturally perform better the second time around regardless of the educational program itself. This threat to internal validity may be termed *testing effect*. It is important to note that testing effects do not always operate to overstate the true effect of a program. Rather, it is possible that pretests may produce such anxiety in individuals that they do much worse on a posttest; thus the effects of a program may be underestimated.

Instrumentation effects. The results obtained may not be valid if the questionnaires administered before the program and after the program were not identical or if the interviewers were not the same or, even if the interviewers were the same, if the questions were asked in a different fashion (perhaps with a different degree of emphasis) from one period to the next. Thus, the program results would be due to changes in the measuring instrument or the people involved in administering those instruments. This is referred to as *instrumentation effect*.

Regression artifact effects. Another potential threat to validity concerns the possibility that the people selected for the program may have had unusually low—or high—levels of health knowledge; that is, they may have been selected on the basis of their *extreme scores*. When tested again, their knowledge scores will have tended to *regress toward the mean* regardless of the effect of the program. This is referred to as the *regression artifact effect*.

Two explanations may be given to obtain a clearer understanding of this phenomenon. The first derives from an understanding of the correlation between two tests. The lower the correlation between pretest and posttest scores, the greater the regression toward the mean. In other words, individuals with a particularly low knowledge-of-disease score on the pretest can be expected to do better on the posttest because of imperfect correlation between the two tests. No true change has taken place; rather, the test scores simply show a test-retest correlation less than unity.

The second explanation concerns errors of measurement. The more deviant a set of scores, in the sense of being selected for extremely high or low values, the larger the error measurement they will contain. Intuitively, we know the extremely low scorers have had unusually bad luck (large negative errors), while the extremely high scorers have had unusually good luck (large positive error). But because such luck is not likely to hold up over time, we expect on a posttest to find the low scores improving somewhat on the average and the high scores declining somewhat.

A graphic illustration of the regression phenomenon, taken from Campbell and Stanley,[1] is presented in Fig. 4, A. In the example, the correlation between the pretest and posttest scores is .50, with no change in group mean (10.0) or variance. Examination of those with pretest scores of 7 reveals somewhat better posttest scores of 7, 8, 9, and 10, and on the average "regressed" halfway to the group mean of 10.0, resulting in a mean of 8.5. In similar fashion, the few individuals who scored 13 on the pretest reveal scores of 10, 11, 12, and 13 on the posttest, showing generally poorer results, and on average "regressed" halfway to the group mean from 13 to 11.5 (the group mean being 10.0). This regression to the mean phenomenon is shown further in Fig. 4, *B* and *C*. As can be seen, these changes are not due to the effect of the program being tested, but rather are the result of the imperfect correlation between pretest and posttest scores.

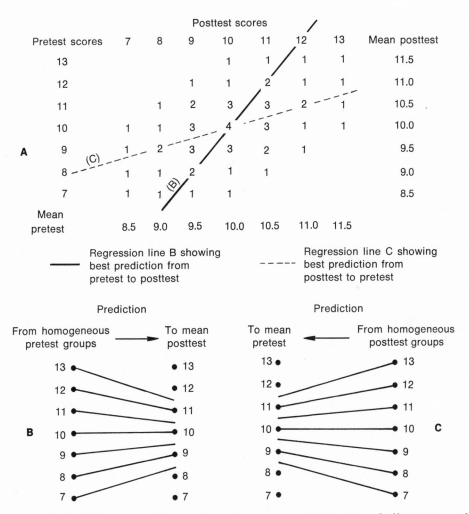

Fig. 4. A–C, Illustration of regression phenomenon. (From Campbell, D. T., and Stanley, J. C.: Experimental and quasi-experimental designs for research, Skokic, Ill., 1966, Rand McNally & Co., p. 10.)

It should be noted that the regression effect phenomenon applies only in cases where individuals have been selected *because of their extreme scores.* In such cases, for the reasons indicated above, these individual scores will regress toward the mean of the population from which they were selected. But the regression effect phenomenon does not apply to individuals *not* selected on the basis of their extreme scores, even though it may turn out that they have extreme scores. In other words, such individuals have been selected for *independent reasons* not related to their extreme scores. In such cases, there is less expectation that the group mean will regress from the pretest to the posttest because random or extraneous scores of variance have been allowed to affect the initial scores in both directions (positive as well as negative).

In addition to the threats of testing, instrumentation, and regression, the previously mentioned threats of history and maturation remain. In order to deal with some of these problems, a second colleague suggests that you do away with the pretest (thus eliminating the potential problems of testing, instrumentation, and regression), but at the same time add a comparison group so that the effects of history and maturation might be ruled out. The suggestion might be diagrammed as follows:

$$\frac{X \quad O_1}{O_2}$$

Here, X again indicates the health education program, O_1 indicates the posttest measure of knowledge in the group which had the program, and O_2 indicates the same measure of knowledge in the group which did not have the program. The solid line indicates that this second group is a *comparison group only* and not a true control group, which would be created by random allocation of subjects to experimental and nonexperimental groups. The design your colleague has suggested may be termed the *static group comparison.*

In considering this design, clearly you can ignore the effects of testing, instrumentation, and regression since these potential threats to validity all refer to the administration of a pretest. You can usually rule out the effects of history as well, since any events (such as a special television program or newspaper series) which might affect the scores of the treatment group should also affect the scores of the comparison group. In brief, the comparison group as well as the treatment group are both exposed to such historical events and, therefore, any change in the posttest knowledge scores may still be attributed to the effect of the program, since the historical influences were basically the same for each. An exception to this occurs in the case of *intra-session history.* That is, the treatment group may have experienced a set of historical events, by virtue of being in the treatment group, which the comparison group did not. For example, hints may have been suggested to the treatment people that a special program or newspaper series was going to take place or, in the very act of coming together for the educational sessions, the program participants may have had a chance to exchange information about such events while this opportunity was unavailable to the comparison group. In such circumstances, any differences between the two groups might be due to such factors rather than the actual content of the health education program itself.

Selection effects. While you may feel quite comfortable that historical events have been controlled (with the possible exception of intra-session history), you are much less sure of maturation effects. Differences in the posttest knowledge scores could be due to maturation effects present in the treatment group that are not present in the comparison group, or vice versa. This depends on the degree to which the treatment group and comparison group are similar in the characteristics (age, sex, health status, previous health knowledge) which affect program results. Thus, the concern is with selection factors and the problem really involves the interaction of *selection and maturation*. For example, if those receiving the program were in poorer health than the comparison group, then it could be that, if their health continued to deteriorate over the course of the program, they would learn more about their health than would the comparison group, *not* because of the educational program as such, but because of their increased interest and awareness of their deteriorating health condition.

Selection effects can also interact with history to pose a threat to internal validity. This frequently occurs, for example, when there has been a differential selection in regard to ethnic groups. Ethnic groups tend to interpret historical events quite differently and, indeed, may consider certain events as historically important which others do not. If the historical event is in any way thought to be related to program effect, careful attention must be paid to interpreting program results.

In addition to its possible association with maturation effects, *selection* itself is an important source of invalidity in using the static group comparison design. In brief, to the extent that the treatment group and control group are not really equivalent, then the results may be due to the nonequivalent factors, such as differences in age, sex, and health status, rather than the educational program. For example, the group receiving the educational program may have scored better than the comparison group because the participants were significantly older, had more illness, and therefore had the opportunity to learn more about various diseases than the younger comparison group. Differences obtained could thus be attributed to differences in the age composition of the two groups and not to the program itself.

Differential attrition. Another threat to the internal validity of this design involves *attrition* — that is, differential rates of people dropping out of the two groups. Attrition is generally not a problem for designs involving only one measurement period but could arise in cases where a comparison group was chosen to be as similar as possible to an experimental group to receive a program at some future time. By the time the program is put into effect and critical observations made, people could have dropped out of the program or, in the case of a comparison group, left the area. For example, even if the two groups were originally identical on key variables such as age or sex, if a greater percentage of older people dropped out of the experimental group, then the results, following the reasoning mentioned above concerning the relationship between age and experience with disease, would tend to favor the comparison group. In summary, the three designs considered so far (one-shot case study, one group pretest-posttest, and static group comparison) all suffer from at least two or more threats to internal validity. These threats along with the designs to which they apply are summarized in Table 3. Table 4 provides the same information organized according to the designs themselves.

Threats to external validity

At this point in your analysis of the health education program, you have concluded that the earlier results and interpretation of those results are not

Table 3. Summary of threats to internal validity

Potential threat	Relevant to these designs	
1. *History*		
Discrete events external to the	One-shot case study	X O
subjects	One group pretest-posttest	$O_1 X O_2$
2. *Maturation*		
Events occurring within subjects as a	One-shot case study	O X
systematic function of time	One group pretest-posttest	$O_1 X O_2$
3. *Testing*		
Providing a pretest which may affect	One group pretest-posttest	$O_1 X O_2$
subjects in either a positive or negative		
fashion such as to influence results		
4. *Instrumentation*		
Changes in the measuring instrument	One group pretest-posttest	$O_1 X O_2$
or those administering the measuring		
instrument which might cause changes		
in the program results		
5. *Regression artifacts*		
Where subjects have been selected on	One group pretest-posttest	$O_1 X O_2$
the basis of their extreme scores,		
program results will be affected by fact		
that these extreme scores will have		
naturally regressed toward the mean		
6. *Selection*		
Differences in the composition of	Static group comparison	X O_1
subjects making up the treatment and		———
comparison groups		O_2
7. *Attrition*		
Differential drop-out of subjects	Static group comparison	X O_1
between the treatment and comparison		———
group		O_2
8. *Selection-maturation interaction*		
Differences in maturation effects due	Static group comparison	X O_1
to selection differences in the		———
composition of subjects making up the		O_2
treatment and comparison group		
9. *Selection-history interaction*		
Differences in exposure to or	Static group comparison	X O_1
interpretation of historical events due		———
to selection differences in the		O_2
composition of subjects making up the		
treatment and comparison group		

Table 4. Potential threats to internal validity*

Design	History	Maturation	Testing	Instrumentation	Regression artifacts	Selection	Attrition	Selection-maturation interaction	Selection-history interaction
1. One-shot case study X O	x†	x							
2. One group pretest-posttest $O_1 X O_2$	x	x	x	x	x				
3. Static group comparison $X \; \underline{O_1}$ O_2						x	x	x	x

*Adapted from Campbell, D. T., and Stanley, J. C.: Experimental and quasi-experimental designs for research, Skokie, Ill., 1966, Rand McNally & Company, p. 8.
†Presence of potential threat to internal validity.

valid. Furthermore, alternative ways of evaluating the program, such as introducing a pretest or introducing a comparison group, while solving some problems, simultaneously create additional threats to internal validity. Without internally valid results, you are well aware that the findings cannot be generalized to other clinic patients and that new programs cannot be based on this evaluation. To the extent that any of the threats to internal validity are present, external validity is threatened as well. However, even if you were able to obtain internally valid results by randomly allocating patients to a treatment and control group (thereby creating a true experimental design), a number of factors might constrain the extent to which results could be generalized. The four most important to consider are (1) the interaction of selection and the treatment program, (2) the interaction of testing and the treatment program, (3) situational or "reactive" effects, and (4) multiple treatment or "combined" treatment effects.

Selection-treatment interaction. The interaction of selection and treatment refers to the possibility that the program results may be applicable only to that population from which the experimental and control groups were chosen. For example, with random selection and allocation of patients to treatment and control groups, the results of the health education program would be internally valid to your particular hospital and generalizable to all outpatients which your hospital serves but may *not* be generalizable to other hospitals *unlike* your own which serve a *different population* of patients. In brief, what works in one hospital may not work in another because of different population characteristics. Furthermore, what works for one hospital during a particular time period *may not apply in another time period,* particularly to a hospital unlike your own in the type of population served. Ideally, in order to increase the *statistical generalizability* of program findings, you would have to sample a number of different types of hospitals with different populations and randomly allocate patients to treatment and control groups. (For a further discussion of such designs, see Campbell and Stanley and related readings suggested at the end of this chapter.) Alternatively, a number of quasiexperimental designs to be discussed later in the chapter might be used.

Statistical generalizability, sometimes referred to as the "statistical span,"[2] is not the only consideration involved. When there is little knowledge in a given area and the issue is important, it makes sense to suggest to others that one's particular program results *may* be applicable in a wide variety of other settings and situations so as to encourage further testing and replication in those settings. This is referred to as "subject matter span"[2] and is usually much broader than strict "statistical span" will permit.

Testing-treatment interaction. The interaction of treatment and testing (where a pretest has been administered) refers to the fact that the program results may be generalized to other groups only when a pretest is also given. For example, in the case of the health education program other similar hospitals with similar patients may wish to use your posttest scores as norms of what to expect. But actual implementation of the program in these hospitals may result in scores lower than the "norms." This may be due not to program failure but rather to the fact that a *pretest* was not given before the program was introduced. Such an interaction is most likely to occur when the pretest is very sensitive to program participants, causing them to be particularly influenced (either positively or negatively) by the program to follow. What little evidence exists suggests that such effects are small.[2] Nevertheless, such a possibility should be evaluated in advance when contemplating the design of a particular program. Of course, such an interaction can be ruled out by eliminating the pretest or by adding additional control groups. Both of these situations are described later.

Situation effects. Situational effects refer to the existence of multiple factors associated with the experiment itself. These include such factors as the personnel involved in the program, the extent to which the subjects are aware that they are part of an experiment (the "Hawthorne effect"), the newness of the program, and the particular period of time in which the experiment is conducted. For example, returning to our health education example, the results achieved may be due to a particularly charismatic health educator. While the results are internally valid for our particular hospital setting, other settings might not expect to achieve the same effects without a similarly charismatic teacher. Or it might be that our study patients, sensing that they are part of an experiment, may try harder and thereby obtain scores much higher than might be expected in the absence of such an awareness. Or the newness of the program might result in temporary increases in knowledge which, if generalized to other situations, might not hold up over time. Or our program may have been conducted during a period of increased national interest in health education, and we might not expect the same results at some future time period. Finally, if our program has been conducted in a special building (perhaps called the Consumer Health Education Center), we might not expect other hospitals to achieve the same results without such special facilities.

Multiple treatment effects. In Chapter 2 we discussed the growing complexity of many health services programs. What exactly constitutes the treatment program is often not clear. A related problem concerns situations in which subjects are involved in a number of programs either immediately before entering the program to be evaluated or at the same time as the program of interest. In the former case, the particular program results may not be generalizable to other settings because they are in part due to the fact that both experimental and control groups were involved in a previous program prior to the one of interest, while this may not be the case in other settings. For example, some fraction of our health education study patients (both treatment and control groups) may have been previously enrolled in an obesity clinic where they picked up some knowledge of health and disease. In the case where multiple treatments are occurring simultaneously, it is difficult to generalize particular program results to settings in which such multiple treatments may not be occurring. For example, our health education study participants may be a part of several medical care utilization and evaluation studies being conducted by the hospital. Thus, while we may be confident that the health education program produces positive results in our particular setting, it may not do so in other settings lacking a similar variety of simultaneous programs.

While we may be reasonably assured that our health education program has indeed produced internally valid results for our own hospital, the additional issues mentioned above are to be examined when considering whether the program should be adopted by other hospitals or health care organizations. In the following section, various designs for overcoming some of these "external" constraints as well as strengthening internal validity will be discussed.

Evaluation designs
Randomization and sampling

The cornerstone of experimental evaluation designs is the random allocation of subjects to treatment and control groups. Randomization is a powerful tool that increases the probability that treatment and control groups will be alike so that alternative explanations for program results such as selection bias, selection-maturation interaction, and regression artifacts may be ruled out.

Randomization is particularly important when the effects of the program are expected to be *small*. It is important to note that this situation is particularly applicable to health care programs. When the effect of a particular program is expected to be so large as to overwhelm selection biases and variability from group to group, randomization is somewhat less important.

When the *sample size* is small, randomization does not always ensure equivalent treatment and control groups. With small sample sizes it is possible to obtain what might be called a "bad luck" randomization. In such a situation the *precision* of the study can be increased by *matching* individuals before random assignment.

There are two basic types of matching—*precision control* and *frequency distribution control*. Precision control refers to pairwise matching in which, for each individual in the treatment group, an individual with the same combination of categories of background variables is selected for the comparison group. For example, if age, sex, and education were the background variables of interest in the health education program, then one would match for all three of these variables *in combination*—for example, females between 21 and 30, with 12 or more years of education. This type of matching usually requires a large number of subjects because of the difficulty in finding individuals who match on all three categories; it is therefore less useful in ensuring equivalence with small sample sizes.

More relevant in such cases is frequency distribution control, which attempts to gain the advantage of matching for several variables without discarding as many subjects as is necessary with precision control. With frequency distribution control, the two groups are equated for each of the matching variables *separately* but not in combination. Thus, the number of females would be matched in the two groups, the number of individuals between 21 and 30, and the number of individuals with 12 or more years of education. But there is no assurance that the combination of sex, age, and education are the same in each group. After the individuals have been matched, using either precision control or frequency distribution control, individuals from each pair may then be randomly allocated to treatment and control groups. This not only helps to ensure the equivalence of the two groups but also strengthens the inferences which can be drawn from the data since the treatment-control group comparisons can be made over many pairs.

Given the obvious advantages of randomization one might wonder why it is not employed more frequently in evaluating health care programs. The major reasons appear to center around ethical and administrative concerns, with the former being the more important. Opponents of randomization contend that it is unethical to withhold treatment or services from groups of people who might benefit from them or, in contrast, it is unethical to *expose* people to a particular experimental treatment or program that might be harmful to them. Proponents of randomization, on the other hand, argue that the number of instances in which it would be unethical to randomize subjects is smaller than generally believed. They note that the withholding of a particular treatment or program exposure does not mean that the control group receives no services at all. In many cases, for example, drug therapy and other treatment activities, they continue to receive the best treatment currently available. The purpose of the evaluation itself is to determine whether the new program or treatment is really better than what is currently available. Proponents would argue that it is far better to conduct some carefully designed evaluative trials with the voluntary consent of informed participants to determine the efficiency of a new program or treatment than to spend a good deal of money putting the population at large at risk while learning little. Some refer to the latter policy as "fooling around with people."[3]

The primary administrative concerns involve cost and convenience. If a large number of subjects is involved (several hundred or more) the clerical and research assistant costs of carrying out and validating the randomization might be of concern. Perhaps of greater importance is the inconvenience which might be caused to existing organizational members and existing organizational procedures to treat individuals who have been randomly assigned to a particular program rather than simply taking individuals as they appear for treatment.

Such arguments should serve to sensitize future administrators and providers to the issues. Actual decisions must be made on the merit of particular situations and circumstances rather than on abstract considerations. The process essentially involves an answer to the question of whether the potential benefits of randomization outweigh the potential costs. Some variables to be considered in this process include (1) number of people to be potentially affected, (2) seriousness of the problem or issue to which the treatment program is addressed, (3) political importance of the issue, and (4) length of the experimental period, in addition to the specific benefits and costs associated with the evaluation itself. In general, the greater the number of people in society for whom the program is eventually intended, the more serious the problem or issue being addressed, the greater the political consequences (in particular costs) of implementing the program on a wide basis, and the larger the time period required for study, then the greater are the benefits associated with random assignment of subjects during the evaluation study.

When randomization is not possible (on ethical, administrative, or political grounds) the earlier mentioned matching techniques of precision control or frequency distribution control should be used to attempt to equate the treatment and control groups. That is, in addition to strengthening randomization, matching techniques can be used as a substitute for randomization. Alternatively, data analysis techniques are available to statistically remove the effects of differences between the two groups. However, it is becoming increasingly evident that neither matching nor statistical adjustments are very good substitutes for true random allocation. For example, in an evaluation of educational experiments employing non-randomized designs, Campbell and Boruch have found systematic underestimation of program effects.[4] Thus, when possible, random allocation of subjects should be employed; what should be done when this is not possible is discussed later in this chapter.

This discussion has focused on the random allocation of subjects to treatment and control groups. Randomization not only controls for most threats to internal validity but also increases external validity by ruling out selection-treatment interaction effects. However, external validity (the extent to which the evaluated program's results can be generalized to other settings and situations) also depends heavily on the nature of the population from which the study subjects (both treatment group and control group) were sampled. In order to increase the probability of a representative sample, *random sampling* is necessary. A *simple random sample* assures everyone from a defined population an equal chance of being selected. In the case of the health education program, we might obtain lists of all people in our target area or all people who had used the outpatient clinic during the previous year and then, using a random numbers table, randomly select individuals for the study. In the same process we could, of course, randomly allocate individuals to the treatment and control groups. From a sampling theory viewpoint, it is important to note that internally valid program findings can only be generalized to the population from which the sample was drawn and to other populations possessing these exact same characteristics.

In many cases, a simple random sample will suffice. But in some cases we may wish to increase the precision of our sample or obtain the same precision for less cost by drawing a *stratified random sample*. In other cases, again for cost and convenience considerations, we may wish to draw a *cluster sample or areal multi-stage stratified sample*.

A stratified random sample is one which first divides a population into a number of strata; then a random sample is selected within each stratum. Such samples can be drawn on a *proportionate* basis in which an equal percentage is selected from each stratum, or on a *disproportionate* basis in which a greater percentage is drawn from some strata than others. For example, if we wished to study hospital inpatient utilization we could divide patients according to age and sex categories (strata) and take a selected percentage (for example, 20 percent) of patients in each category. This is an example of a proportionate stratified sample in that the same proportion of patients would be taken from each stratum or category.

Disproportional stratified random sampling is particularly appropriate when the variable under study is highly skewed. For example, a few large hospitals in an area might account for a large percentage of all area admissions. In such cases, one might wish to take a 100 percent sample in those hospitals while selecting proportionately fewer hospitals in other bed-size categories.

Stratified random samples increase the precision of a sample by making sure that certain characteristics of interest, such as age, sex, and bed size, will be well represented in the sample.

The main purpose of a cluster sample is to reduce the costs of collecting data. For example, if we wanted to collect data on 200 households in a town of 20,000, we could take a 1 percent random sample. But this would spread the interviewers out over the entire town. An alternative would be to concentrate the data collection in a few parts of town. For example, if the town were divided into 400 areas of 50 households each, we could select at random four areas in the town (1 in 100) and include all the households within those areas in our sample. The overall probability of selection remains unchanged, but by selecting clusters of households the cost of collecting the data has been reduced and convenience increased.

Areal multi-stage stratified sampling is used mainly in large-scale social surveys and large social experiments. First, geographic areas are randomly selected based on variables of interest such as size, location, density, and so on. Then within these areas certain census tracts are randomly selected. All the households within these census tracts are then listed out and certain households are selected randomly to participate in the experiment or social survey. Again, major advantages are in terms of cost and convenience.

While most administrators, planners, and providers will be involved primarily in relatively small-scale discrete program evaluation efforts for which simple random and stratified random samples will suffice, some will become involved in larger scale efforts (for example, Rand Health Insurance Experiment), and thus some familiarity with sampling techniques relevant to such efforts is useful.

A "true" experimental design

In the evaluation of the health education program, you found a number of weaknesses in the design as well as in alternatives suggested by colleagues. (See Table 3 for a summary). Recognizing the importance of having a control group and the process of randomization, you realize that stronger inferences regarding program results could have been drawn if patients, after the initial pretest of health knowledge, had been randomly allocated to a treatment group (those to receive health education program) and a control group (those not to receive the program). Such a design is commonly called a *pretest-posttest control group design*. It may be diagrammed as follows:

$$\frac{R \ O_1 \ X \ O_2}{R \ O_3 \quad O_4}$$

Here, R indicates random allocation of patients, O_1 and O_2 indicate the pretest and posttest for the treatment group, X indicates the treatment group, O_3 and O_4 indicate the pretest and posttest for the control group, and the dashed line indicates that the group below the line is a true control group due to randomization of subjects. This design generally guards against all threats to internal validity except differential experimental attrition (that is, a greater number of program dropouts or deletions in one group than the other). Except for the possibility of intrasession history, *historical events* are controlled for since any event which affects the treatment group also affects the control group. *Maturation* is controlled for through the random allocation of patients to both groups. There is no reason to expect one group to generate maturational effects any differently from the other group. *Testing* is controlled for in that both groups are exposed to an identical pretest. If the pretest did have any sensitizing effect, it should have occurred for both groups. *Instrumentation* is controlled for to the extent that the tests used at time O_1 and O_3 are identical and that those used at time O_2 and O_4 are identical. If interviewers are used, it is important that they be randomly assigned to the treatment and control groups and that they be *unaware* of which is the treatment and which the control group. Furthermore, the *same* interviewer who conducted the pretest interview with a particular group of patients should conduct the posttest interview with the same group of patients. *Regression effects* are controlled for by the random allocation of patients to the treatment and control groups. Even if we wanted to examine the effects of the program on those people with very low levels of health knowledge, internal validity would be assured as long as the sample of individuals from the "low knowledge" population was *randomly* allocated to the treatment and control groups. Whatever regression to the mean effects might occur would be expected to be *similar* for both groups, thus permitting program inferences to be drawn regarding any differences which might be observed between the treatment and control groups. *Selection* is obviously controlled to the extent that randomization has assured the equivalence of the two groups prior to introduction of the program. As mentioned, this assurance is greater the greater the number of people involved in the study. Different rates of *attrition* between treatment and control groups are *never controlled for* by any design. But with a control group, it becomes possible to determine the extent of the differential attrition and assess its likely impact on overall program results. For example, if a greater number of elderly people dropped out of the control group in the health education study than in the treatment group, one might randomly delete the scores of an equivalent number of elderly from the treatment group and reanalyze the program findings. To some extent this can also be done with comparison groups (groups to whom a nonrandomized treatment group is being compared), but it is more dangerous because one has no assurance that the two groups were the same at the beginning. Finally, any interaction effects involving selection and maturation, selection and history, and so on are once again controlled for to the extent that randomization has indeed assured the equivalence of the two groups.

Thus, if in using the above design we found that the group receiving the program had a statistically significant higher increase in health knowledge than the control group, we would be quite confident that this increase was indeed due to our health education program and not to some other factor; this, of course, is the entire issue of internal validity. But we would be on less firm ground in suggesting that the same beneficial results might be achieved in other hospitals or ambulatory care clinics or even in other units of our own hospital. Leaving aside the fact that one can only generalize to populations similar to the one from which the study sample was selected and the problems of situational and multiple treatment effects previously discussed, the major external validity limitation of the pretest-posttest control group design is the possibility of an interaction between the pretest and the treatment. In the context of the present example, the improvement in health knowledge may only take place in combination with a pretest being given. Thus, other settings implementing the program without a pretest may not achieve the same results.

If high importance is being given to the external validity of program results (such as for a study group hospital which is part of a multi-unit chain to which the ownership wishes to generalize the results) and testing-treatment interaction is expected to be an issue, a couple of alternative designs may be used to deal with the problem. The first is simply to drop the pretest. This may be diagrammed as

$$R \quad X \quad O_1$$
$$R \quad \quad O_2$$

and referred to as the *posttest-only control group design*. If the O_1 average score is statistically significantly greater than the O_2 mean score, then this can be validly attributed to the effects of the program and, in addition, other settings of like characteristics (situational and treatment effects aside) might also expect to achieve the same results. This design depends crucially on the fact that randomization has indeed made the two groups equivalent at the beginning of the study.

An alternative to deleting the pretest is to actually try to remove the effects of the pretest on program results. This may be done by adding two more groups of subjects to the study, diagrammed as follows:

$$R \, O_1 \, X \, O_2$$
$$R \, O_3 \quad O_4$$
$$R \quad X \, O_5$$
$$R \quad \quad O_6$$

This is called, after its originator, the *Solomon Four-Group Design*.[5] The two new groups are designated as O_4 and O_6; neither group is given a pretest, but O_5 receives the treatment program while O_6 does not. In brief, the bottom half of the design constitutes the posttest-only design just described, while the upper half constitutes the classic pretest-posttest control group design. In combination they allow for the effects of possible pretest-treatment interactions to be assessed. The most relevant comparisons are the O_2 versus O_1 results, O_2 versus O_4, O_5 versus O_6, and O_5 versus O_3. If $O_2 - O_1 > O_4 - O_3$, we know the program has had a beneficial impact but are not sure about the testing-treatment interaction issue. But if $O_5 > O_6$, then we are reasonably confident we can ignore testing-treatment interaction as limiting the generalizability or external validity of our findings. Furthermore, the extent of testing-treatment interaction may be measured by comparing the differences between O_4 scores and O_6 scores, which indicate the effect of testing for those not receiving the program, and the difference between O_2 and O_5 scores, which indicate the effect of testing for those receiving the program. If these effects are approximately the same ($O_4 - O_6 \approx O_2 - O_5$), then we can conclude that no testing-treatment interaction effects exist. If they are statistically significantly different ($O_4 - O_6 \neq O_2 - O_5$), then we conclude that there is an interaction between testing and treatment, and it is measured by the magnitude of the inequality in the two difference scores.

The major limitation of the Solomon Four-Group Design is the cost and inconvenience of including two additional study groups. In many cases, there will not be a large enough number of subjects to be able to create four randomly allocated groups. In these circumstances one is left with the posttest-only control group design which, although unable to measure the extent of testing-treatment interaction, effectively eliminates it as a possible threat to external validity.

These designs permit the strongest inferences to be drawn regarding the extent to which the effects observed may really be attributed to the program under evaluation. To the extent that political, administrative, and ethical conditions permit, such designs should be employed. This is particularly the case if the issue at hand is highly salient and likely to affect large numbers of people, and if key groups in society are divided as to the usefulness of implementing or extending a program on a wide scale. The Salk vaccine trials serve as a good example from the biomedical area, and the Rand Health Insurance Experiment from the health services delivery area. If the conditions of salience, large numbers of people, and controversy do not exist, then less rigorous designs may suffice. This may clearly be necessary if one is faced with various constraints, for example, administrative (money and time limitations), political (fear of negative results), or ethical (community pressure over withholding of services). In such situations it is important to be able to creatively analyze a number of possible alternative strategies for program evaluation which, while not containing the rigor of a controlled experimental trial, will eliminate as many sources of competing explanations as possible. Examples of five such designs are discussed in the following section.

Quasi-experimental designs

A number of designs which do not involve random allocation of subjects to treatment and control groups may nevertheless approximate some of the advantages of a true experimental design. These are referred to as *quasi-*experimental designs precisely because they do not involve random allocation of subjects to treatment and control groups. The pros and cons of five designs relevant to health services program evaluation are described next.

Time series design. Suppose you wanted to evaluate the impact of a statewide cervical cancer screening program on the number of Pap smears completed for a defined group (for example, women over 16 years of age residing in families with incomes at or below 200 percent of federal poverty guidelines). Assume that political and ethical considerations prevent you from randomly assigning individuals to a treatment and control group. Furthermore, you are not given enough funds to collect data from a matched compari-

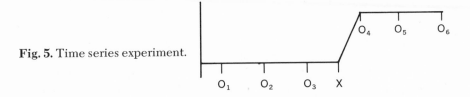

Fig. 5. Time series experiment.

son group state. A simple pretest-posttest design can be devised but you are aware that any differences obtained might also be explained by historical effects (public media coverage) or maturational effects (change in fertility rates). How can you guard against these particular sources of invalidity within the constraints of the situation?

One possibility is to obtain *multiple measures* both before and after introduction of the cervical screening program. This is shown in Fig. 5; O_1, O_2, and O_3 represent measures of the percentage of women screened in the 3 consecutive years before the program went into effect, X represents the introduction of the program, and O_4, O_5, and O_6 represent measures of the percentage of women screened in the 3 years after the program was in effect. This is commonly referred to as a *time series experiment.*

The primary advantages of this design over the single pretest-posttest design are its control of maturational effects and partial control of history effects. This is due to the effect of having multiple measures before introduction of the program. For example, if the change in the percentage screened from period O_3 to O_4 were due to changes in fertility rates, this effect should have also been observed in the earlier time periods, that is, between O_1 and O_2 and between O_2 and O_3. Similarly, if the O_3 to O_4 jump can be explained by a historical event such as extensive public media coverage of cervical cancer, this should also have been true in earlier time periods (O_1 to O_2 and O_2 to O_3) when similar historical events must have also occurred. In order for history to be a plausible alternative explanation of O_3 to O_4 changes, the event would have to be unique and specific to that time period only and not to immediately preceding time periods.

The multiple time series design is most useful when evaluating programs which are *not subject to cyclical or seasonal shifts.* For example, a recent evaluation of a Connecticut traffic safety program incorrectly attributed a decline in auto fatalities to the effect of the program, when in fact the fatalities for the year in question simply reflected a cyclical trend.[6] In other words, the program was introduced at a point in the cycle in which traffic fatalities were high and due to fall naturally during the next time period with or without the program. This phenomenon is illustrated in Fig. 6, *A.* When such cyclical shifts are present, or at least suspected, it is necessary that the observation of recurrent periods be sufficiently frequent to include the different stages of the cycle. One can then compare entire cycles, as shown in Fig. 6, *B,* to see if the *overall* trend or cycle after introduction of the program is different from the *overall* trend before the program. Fig. 6, *B,* also illustrates the importance of having multiple measures after the program not only to evaluate overall shifts

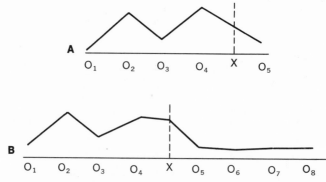

Fig. 6. **A,** Time series design with cyclical or seasonal event—conclusion that program has had an impact is incorrect. **B,** Conclusion that program has had an impact is consistent with the observations.

in cycles but to assess the permanence and stability of program impact over time, regardless of whether cycles are present.

Where pretests are given (for example, in our earlier mentioned health education program), this design also enables *testing effects* to be critically studied because of the multiple measures involved. Generally, testing will not be a threat to internal validity because if O_3 to O_4 changes were due to testing effects, they should have also been observed during O_1 to O_2 and O_2 to O_3 time periods.

However, problems can arise with *instrumentation* effects if the "instruments" being used are observers or interviewers. The observers or interviewers may experience boredom or fatigue over the different observation periods. Or if the observers are aware of when the program was introduced they may unwittingly bias their recording in favor of the program having a positive impact.

Regression effects are generally not a problem with time series designs because such effects generally disappear over time. Thus, if women with an unusually low Pap smear completion rate had been deliberately selected, we would expect that their rate would naturally regress upward toward the mean by the next time period and by the third time period before introduction of the program will have demonstrated some stability. Again, as noted earlier, it is important to make sure that one is not dealing with a highly cyclical phenomenon.

Since there are no control or comparison groups, *selection* is not a factor. While *attrition* is not controlled, it can be readily assessed by examining the rate and composition of dropouts (for example, people leaving the state) during the O_3 to O_4 period and comparing it to the rate and composition of dropouts in the other time periods.

The program, of course, may interact with selection and testing factors to limit external validity along with any limitations which may be present due to situational or multiple treatment effects. There is no substitute for replication of time series evaluations in other settings before confidence can be placed in the generalizability of results.

It is also important to note that *prospective* time series designs are vastly superior to retrospective assessments because one is able to determine precisely the time at which the program is introduced. With retrospective, after-the-fact assessments, it is sometimes difficult to be exactly sure of when a particular program was introduced. For example, if one wished to assess the impact of expanded-duty dental auxiliaries on dental productivity, it would be easier to do this prospectively, as dentists hire auxiliaries, than to attempt a retrospective assessment, which would be dependent on memory recall of previous hiring practices.

While history and instrumentation effects must be closely monitored, the time series design controls for many of the remaining threats to validity. It is particularly appropriate to use in evaluating programs for which data on the relevant outcome measures have been collected for a number of previously consecutive time periods.

Multiple time series. The *multiple time series* operates on the same principles described for the single time series above except a comparison group, matched with the treatment group to the extent possible, is added. It may be diagrammed as follows:

$$\frac{O_1\ O_2\ O_3\ X\ O_4\ O_5\ O_6}{O_7\ O_8\ O_9\qquad O_{10}\ O_{11}\ O_{12}}$$

Multiple observations are collected on both groups both before and after the introduction of the program. The major advantage of the multiple time series is that it provides a somewhat *stricter control for historical effects*. For example, if the shift from O_3 to O_4 is due to a historical event occurring exactly at the time period, then we might expect the same effect to occur in the comparison group between the O_9 and O_{10} observation points. Thus, if the shift from O_3 to O_4 is still greater than the shift from O_9 to O_{10}, we might safely attribute it to the effect of the program. Our confidence in such an attribution would of course depend on the extent to which the treatment and comparison groups were really similar. In addition, the greater the similarity of the two groups the more confident we can be in ruling out selection-history, selection-maturation, and selection-instrumentation interaction effects.

A detailed example of a multiple time series design for evaluating the impact of a cervical cancer screening program on the rate of Pap smears completed is presented in the Appendix.

Nonequivalent comparison group. The basic idea behind the *nonequivalent comparison group* design has already been introduced. It is similar to the pretest-posttest control group design discussed earlier, except subjects are not randomly allocated to a treatment group and control group. Instead, a second group is chosen which is as similar as possible to the treatment group. It is similar to the multiple time series design described above, except there is only one pretest and posttest observation rather than multiple observations. The nonequivalent comparison group design may be diagrammed as follows:

$$\frac{O_1\ X\ O_2}{O_3\qquad O_4}$$

The lack of Rs indicates that no randomization has occurred, and the dashed lines indicate that O_3 to O_4 measurements involve a comparison group and not a true control group.

This design is frequently employed in situations which start out as a true pretest-posttest control group evaluation but, for various reasons, randomization had to be abandoned. An interesting case is described below.

The problems of providing appropriate health care for elderly and seriously handicapped individuals in our society are well-known. The needs for long-term care virtually ensure that the process will be expensive and that high levels of satisfaction on either side of the health care system will be difficult to achieve. Nonetheless, it is clear that the system that has evolved over the years is not as satisfactory as it could be and is not working as well as it should. Elderly individuals are too often institutionalized or given degrees of care beyond that really needed by them because there is not a satisfactory alternative. There is also good reason to believe that institutionalization itself can have detrimental effects on the health and welfare of elderly individuals and handicapped persons. What appears to be required is a system of care for these individuals that does not expose them to levels of care beyond their actual needs, which does not make them unduly dependent, and for which costs can be contained. It is equally clear, however, that elderly individuals and handicapped individuals probably require special access to the health system because of the spatial immobilities.

The Fall River (Massachusetts) Housing Authority in collaboration with the Department of Housing and Urban Development (HUD) developed a plan for establishing a medically-oriented housing project that would be a free-standing apartment house specially designed for geriatric and handicapped patients. It would be located in close proximity to a hospital and be connected to it by a tunnel so that there would be access to health care in all kinds of weather and all times of the day or night without great inconvenience or personal risk. An apartment building containing 210 units was actually financed and built by HUD along these lines.

There is an obvious need to determine whether a housing project of the type described here has a desirable impact on the health and welfare of the individuals for whom it is provided. Apartment buildings do not come cheap, and unless they are shown to be effective, they can obviously be a waste of money. In addition, there is the risk that scarce resources will be diverted into useless activities, and also, that attention will be diverted from the persistent, continuing problems of this population of individuals. Consequently, an evaluation research scheme was built into the plans for the Fall River Project. The original plans called for the development of a list of eligible individuals who would then be assigned randomly either to live in this housing project or to remain in whatever housing they occupied at the time. The rationale for this procedure was that the housing available would be a scarce resource. It was believed that there would not be enough apartment units for the people who would want to occupy them and, consequently, some form of lottery or serial assignment was proposed to allocate the housing units available to a portion of the individuals actually eligible for them. *Unfortunately, from the standpoint of the research however, the initial response to the availability of the housing units was not as great as anticipated and the project did not fill up as rapidly as expected. The result of this was that HUD put a great deal of pressure on the housing authority to fill the vacant units. The units were thus filled, frustrating the original design involving randomization.* Although the investigators involved in this project were disheartened by these early problems, they were able to recoup to a considerable degree by developing a comparison group consisting of individuals who were carefully matched on a great many variables with the occupants of the housing authority. Their health status could then be compared with that of the project group.

This project has been going on for a period of almost five years now, and the results are beginning to be evident. There was an early indication that perhaps the mortality rates of the experimentally housed might be lower than that of the comparison group, but the findings seem not to have persisted. However, what has happened is that individuals in the comparison group have had to be placed into various kinds of extended care facilities at an earlier time than the individuals in the medically-oriented housing complex.

If medically-oriented housing is shown to be desirable in terms of the outcomes it produces and to have desirable social impact, this research project would have important implications for current policy at Federal and local levels aimed at the establishment of various alternative care facilities such as skilled nursing homes and the like. Rather than putting money into these extended care facilities which keep elderly persons in unneeded dependent states, it may be better that comparable funds should be invested in providing adequate housing in proximity to medical services so that elderly and handicapped individuals could maintain themselves for longer periods of time as independent community members. Such housing would not necessarily have to be connected by tunnels to a hospital for it could be built in close proximity to medical clinics and group practice settings.[7]

In this example, the investigators relied on matching to ensure the comparability of the two groups. As previously indicated by Campbell and Boruch,[4] this by no means ensures that true program effects can be estimated. But perhaps more pertinent are the limitations involved when the treatment group is composed of individuals who have *volunteered* for the program. In seeking a comparison group one may be able to match on basic demographic characteristics and other variables but there always remain the motivational differences associated with the fact that the treatment group has volunteered for the program while the comparison group has not. In this case, the evaluation may be subject to *selection-history, selection-maturation,* or *selection-testing* interactions which serve as compelling explanations for whatever program results might be found. For example, the individuals who volunteered may be more enthusiastic about the program, which may result in their (1) being exposed to different historical events, (2) experiencing accelerated learning, or (3) being more sensitive to pretest measurement than members of the "matched" group.

Even though matching has been employed, the nonequivalent comparison group design may still be subject to *regression effects.* Campbell and Stanley provide the example of applicants for a therapy program who are "matched" with a comparison group so as to bring about equivalence of pretest self-esteem scores.[1] But it is important to realize that among the matched comparison group are some extremely low scores which on the posttest will regress to a more normal group average and achieve higher self-esteem, thus making it less likely that a significant effect of the therapy program will be shown. Deniston and Rosenstock found similar regression effect problems in their evaluation of a rheumatoid arthritis treatment program.[8] Such limitations as selection-interaction effects and regression effects are much less likely to be serious problems *when two more or less natural groups* (who are seeking the program or are eligible for the program) are available, and one can simply decide who is to receive the program first. The group to receive the program first becomes the treatment group and the other group, matched for the characteristics of the treatment group, becomes the comparison group. In this fashion there are no critical motivational differences of self-selection between the two groups, and thus selection interaction and regression effects are essentially controlled. However, such situations are not always so simple. For example, some of those selected to enter the program may change their minds and not enter. In such cases, the selection differences between the treatment and comparison group will continue to exist. One possible way of dealing with this problem is to delete from the comparison group those individuals with background characteristics similar to those who chose not to enter the program. However, in many cases background characteristics may not particularly distinguish those who chose not to enter the program from those who did.

In summary, the greater the degree of similarity between the treatment and comparison groups (including self-selection factors), the greater the degree of confidence which can be placed in the results of a nonequivalent comparison group design. Any attempts to explain away posttest differences between the treatment and comparison group as not being due to the program must be related to specific selection differences that distinguish the two groups. This design is most useful to program administrators and providers to the extent that it is possible to control who gets the program first. The design is, of course, subject to the usual limitations previously discussed regarding external validity.

Recurrent institutional cycle: a "patched-up" design. Patched-up designs emphasize the need for program administrators, providers, and evaluators to adapt their evaluation to the changing circumstances of program operation. As the program progresses it may be possible to rule out several threats to validity by adding various features to the design. This is particularly the case if some event, activity, or program is being presented to a new group of people on a somewhat regular basis. Such situations are frequent in the case of health care programs. Examples include enrollment periods for health maintenance organizations (HMOs) and prepaid group practices, acceptance periods for renal dialysis and other high technology treatment involving queues, residency programs for medical students and other health professionals, and, at a micromanagement level, employee orientation programs. In these cases it becomes possible to compare the results from those already in or exposed to the program with those about to enter the program. This is commonly referred to as the *recurrent institutional cycles design.*

The main part of this design may be diagrammed as follows:

$$\begin{array}{c} \text{X } O_1 \\ \overline{\phantom{\text{X}}} \quad \overline{O_2 \text{ X } O_3} \end{array}$$

It is important to note that O_1 represents a measurement of people who have been exposed to the program at the same time that another group of people about to enter the program are being measured. The various features of this design may be illustrated by the Seattle Prepaid Health Care Project.[9]

From February, 1971, through January, 1975, a study was conducted to assess, among other things, the impact on health status (perceived health status, disability days, functional limitations, and so on) of providing comprehensive medical benefits at zero price to a group of low-income Model Cities individuals. Since program participants were chosen based on enrollment criteria (primarily income levels) it was not possible to randomly allocate individuals to treatment and control groups. Because it was an ongoing program it was not possible to select a single comparison group, nor was it possible to employ a time series or multiple time series design because multiple measures of individuals' health status in years prior to the study did not exist. Instead, it was believed possible to employ the *recurrent institutional cycle design* in which the health status of people in the program after the first year of enrollment could be compared with the health status (as measured by a baseline interview) of people about to enroll in the program during the second year. These groups would then be followed over time for continuing changes in health status.

It is of interest to note that this design is really three designs in one. The first part of the design (X O_1) is simply a *one-shot case study* subject to all the threats to validity possessed by our earlier mentioned health education program. The second part $(\frac{\text{X } O_1}{O_2})$ is the *static group comparison design* which, as previously noted, is particularly vulnerable to selection and selection-interaction effects. The third part (O_2 X O_3) is the familiar *single group pretest-posttest design* which, as discussed earlier, is subject to threats to validity arising from history, maturation, testing, instrumentation, and selection-interaction effects. But when these three designs are "patched together," a number of threats to validity may be controlled. For example, the static group comparison feature $(\frac{\text{X } O_1}{O_2})$ of the design controls for the effects of history which are not controlled for by the one-shot case study feature (X O_1). In the context of health status assessment, if the health status of the group in the program for a year was significantly better than that of the group just entering the program, it would be difficult to explain away the results on the basis that the group in the program was exposed to different historical events than those not in the program. For example, if a massive influenza epidemic had occurred during the year, it is reasonable to expect it would have affected both groups, and any residual health status differences remaining could still be attributed to the effect of the program.

The static group comparison feature $\left(\dfrac{X\ O_1}{O_2}\right)$ also controls for the effect of testing and instrumentation which is not controlled for by the one group pretest-posttest $(O_2\,X\,O_3)$ feature of the design. Thus, any differences between O_1 and O_2 could not be attributed to interviews preceding the program (which might have sensitized respondents to their health status) because no interviews were conducted.

As long as interviewers were trained identically to administer identical interviews at points O_1 and O_2, instrumentation would appear to be fairly well controlled. However, some problems would still exist because the interviewers would know who had been in the program for a year and who were newly enrolled. Thus, it is possible that the health status questions could be asked in such a way as to elicit more favorable responses from those in the program than from those about to enter.

However, we know that a major problem with the static group comparison concerns the fact that O_1 versus O_2 differences in health status could be due to selection differences between the two groups rather than an effect of the program itself. But, following the second group over time in a single group pretest-posttest context $(O_2\,X\,O_3)$ makes it possible to compare the health status difference between O_3 and O_2. If the health status difference between O_3 and O_2 $(O_3 > O_2)$ is approximately the same as the health status difference between O_1 and O_2 $(O_1 > O_2)$, then we are reasonably safe in ruling out selection effects, because even though the two groups may differ somewhat, they are apparently not affecting the ability of the program to achieve similar results *with each group.* Such a comparison also tends to rule out the possibility that the results might be explained by differential dropout rates in the two groups; that is, even though differential attrition between the two groups may exist, it apparently is not affecting the ability of the program to achieve similar results in each group. The problem becomes more difficult if the O_1 to O_2 and O_2 to O_3 comparisons are *not approximately equal* as would be the case where the O_1 group scores significantly higher on health status than the O_2 group, but the O_3 measurement of the second group shows only slightly improved health status or no change at all. Such findings could be due to selection differences between the two groups; for example, the second group could have *either* a much poorer or a much better initial health status than the first group. That is, the program may have had no effect on the second group because *either* they were in such poor health that the program would not be expected to have much of an effect *or* they were in such good health that the program could not be expected to measurably improve their health. In such cases, statistical adjustment (discussed in Chapter 4) would have to be made before one could draw any inferences concerning program impact.

Thus, the recurrent institutional cycle design controls reasonably well for the effects of history, testing, instrumentation, selection, and attrition. But maturation and regression effects remain as potential alternative explanations of program findings. Maturation effects may not be a serious threat if one is evaluating a program designed to teach people specific skills over a relatively short time period. However, within the context of our current example involving health status, it may indeed be a problem. One way of assessing its effect would be to conduct an analysis of subgroups based on specific age categories or age intervals of interest.

Regression effects may exist if, for example, the first group was enrolled primarily because they were sickest. One would then expect to have better health status on the posttest measure as a function of regression to the mean. In a longitudinal study conducted over several years and several measurement periods it might be possible to eliminate this sort of invalidity by analyzing separately the program results for those enrollment groups selected because of particularly poor health. For these groups, the "regression to the mean" phenomenon would be expected to be similar and any remaining differences might validly be attributed to the impact of the program.

In summary, the recurrent institutional cycle design provides a flexible way of handling some major threats to internal validity and is particularly conducive to settings and circumstances in which new groups of individuals are exposed to ongoing programs. It also offers some control for the interaction of testing and treatment.

Regression-discontinuity analysis. Imagine a teaching hospital wanting to assess whether its residency program did anything more for the doctors selected into the program than for those whom the hospital rejected; or imagine that a foundation wanted to assess the impact of a special career development program. How might they proceed?

The ideal way, of course, would be to randomly assign applicants to a treatment group (those to receive the award, whether it be a fellowship, residency position, or some other award) and a control group (those not to receive the award), and assess the impact on later career achievement. This is recognized as the randomized posttest only control group design $\binom{R \ X \ O_1}{R \ \ \ \ O_2}$. This design would require, for example, that a group of health science students be randomly assigned to two groups upon entry to graduate school. Later on, the school or agency would decide to award one group a 1-year fellowship for advanced study. The career achievement of the two groups would then be measured at subsequent points in time. But since such situations rarely exist, alternatives must be found. One alternative, currently widely practiced, is to simply do an after-the-fact assessment of those who received the award. Program sponsors usually conclude that the program made a positive impact because they found that award recipients are located in "influential" positions, in "prestigious" organizations, doing "significant" work. The problem, of course, is that these individuals would in all probability have been in these same positions or attained similar stature in other positions *without* ever having received the award, because those qualities and characteristics relevant to their being selected for the award are also the same ones most strongly related to later success.

One way of coping with such evaluation issues is to compare the later success of those given the award with those not given the award. This can be done by plotting career achievement scores against the original eligibility criteria scores on which the award was made. An example, adapted from

Campbell and Stanley,[1] is shown in Fig. 7. Career achievement scores are plotted on the Y axis and the scores on which the original award was based are plotted on the X axis. The vertical line indicates the cutoff point. Those with scores at or above this point were given the awards, while those below this point were rejected. Each person's career achievement score is then plotted against that person's corresponding eligibility criteria score; the resulting regression line represents the relationship between the two. If we observe a "discontinuity" in the regression line at the critical cutoff point at which the award was made, we are on reasonably safe ground in stating that the program has had a beneficial effect separate from what the award recipients might have otherwise achieved.

The key to understanding the above statement lies in examining the "jump" or change in the *intercepts* at the award cutoff point. In effect, this involves comparing the scores of those people who did not quite make it (from about 100 to 104 in Fig. 7) with those who just barely made it (from 105 to about 109 in Fig. 7). If the award did not make any difference, then we would not expect much of a change in the career achievement scores of these two very similar groups. The group scoring in the 105 to 109 criteria range might have somewhat higher career achievement scores than the group scoring in the 100 to 104 range simply as a reflection of slightly basic differences in native ability and experiences. This would be observed by a continuation of the regression line. But if instead we observe a marked increase in the career

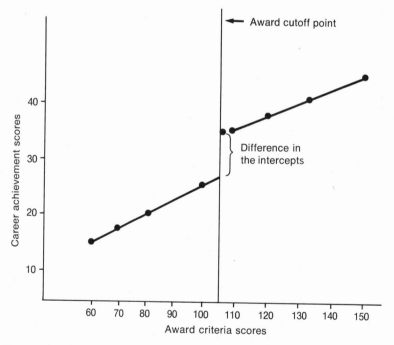

Fig. 7. Regression-discontinuity. (Adapted from Campbell, D. T., and Stanley, J. C.: Experimental and quasi-experimental designs for research, Skokie, Ill., 1966, Rand McNally & Co., p. 62.)

achievement scores of the 105 to 109 criteria group compared with the 100 to 104 criteria group, we have some confidence that the program might indeed have made a beneficial impact independent of the inherent abilities of the award recipients themselves.

This design, or more appropriately "analysis," controls for many of the threats to internal validity and represents a vast improvement over ex post-facto studies or just assuming that the program "did good." *History* and *maturation* would appear to be controlled to the extent that the two groups were considered for the award during the same time period and were followed up for later career achievement over the same time period. *Testing* is controlled in that both groups have been exposed to the test (that is, the initial criteria assessment process). *Instrumentation* problems could exist if the agency which made the award did the follow-up career assessment. In such cases, the award recipients might tend to exaggerate their life achievement while the rejected group might express particularly negative feelings. Or the reverse might occur. The award recipients might tend to play down their accomplishments so as not to attribute them to the award, while the rejected applicants might overexaggerate their accomplishments to indicate to the agency the mistake they had made. Such instrumentation bias is much less of a problem when an independent group does the follow-up assessment. *Selection* and *regression* effects may exist but do not act as a competing explanation of program effects. That is, since the "better" individuals were selected we would expect them to achieve greater success than those not selected, but what we observe at the regression discontinuity point (by examining the intercepts of the two regression lines) is that they perform significantly better—much better than on the basis of selection factors themselves. *Attrition* might be a problem in that one might expect award recipients to be more likely to respond to the follow-up than those not granted the award. Again, if the follow-up is conducted by an independent agency, this is likely to be less of a problem. *Selection-maturation* interaction is controlled in that it would not represent a plausible explanation for a discontinuity of the regression line at the cutoff point for the award.

In regard to external validity, *testing-treatment* interactions are controlled to the extent that the award makes a difference for those people whose scores were closely centered near the cutoff point. *Situational* and *multiple treatment* effects could also pose problems if the award was made during a period of time particularly conducive to later success (a situational effect) or if some of the award recipients also held other awards or received some other form of special treatment at the same time (multiple treatment effect).

In brief, the regression-discontinuity design can control for a number of threats to validity. But it is heavily dependent on the reliability and validity of the criterion scores (the cutoff points) on which the award is based. It also depends on the program making a big enough difference on later "success criteria" so as to be measurable.

Summary. Political, administrative, and ethical considerations frequently exist which preclude use of "true" experimental designs involving random allocation of subjects to treatment and control groups. In such cases, the task is to design an evaluation which will guard against as many of the threats to internal and external validity as possible within the constraints imposed by the political, administrative, and ethical environment of the program being studied. Examples of five such "quasi-experimental" designs have been presented in the preceding section: the single time series, multiple time series, nonequivalent comparison group, recurrent institutional cycle, and regression-discontinuity designs. None of these designs requires random allocation of subjects, and yet, through a variety of mechanisms, they control for a number of threats to internal and external validity. The relative advantages and disadvantages of these designs are summarized in Table 5. The Appendix provides an example of a student evaluation design.

Cost-benefit and cost-effectiveness analysis

The designs that have been described up to this point are intended to show a functional relationship between various inputs or a "treatment" and an outcome or outcomes. As will be discussed in greater detail in Chapter 5, program evaluation results need to be put in a broader policy decision-making context. Sometimes the question of interest to the analyst or program administrator requires a choice among alternative programs in the face of scarce resources. We turn next to a brief description of analytic techniques that build

Table 5. Summary of potential threats to validity for five quasi-experimental designs*

| | \multicolumn{12}{c}{Threats to validity} |
| | \multicolumn{8}{c}{Internal} | \multicolumn{4}{c}{External} |
	History	*Maturation*	*Testing*	*Instrumentation*	*Regression*	*Selection*	*Attrition*	*Interaction of selection and maturation, etc.*	*Interaction of testing and X*	*Interaction of selection and X*	*Reactive arrangements*	*Multiple-X interference*
1. Single time series O_1 O_2 O_3 $O_4 X O_5$ O_6 O_7 O_8	−	+	+	?	+	+	?	+	−	?	?	?
2. Multiple time series O_1 O_2 $O_3 X O_4$ O_5 O_6 O_7 O_8 O_9 O_{10} O_{11} O_{12}	+	+	+	+	+	+	?	+	−	−	?	?
3. Nonequivalent control group design O_1 X O_2 O_3 O_4	+	+	+	+	?	+	?	−	−	?	?	?
4. Institutional cycle design $X O_1$ $O_2 \overline{X O_3}$	+	−	+	+	−	+	?	−	+	?	?	?
5. Regression discontinuity	+	+	+	?	+	+	?	+	+	−	+	+

*Adapted from Campbell, D. T., and Stanley, J. C.: Experimental and quasi-experimental designs for research, Skokie, Ill., 1966, Rand McNally & Company, pp. 40, 56.

on program evaluation results and provide a formal way of evaluating alternatives.

Although the application of cost-benefit analysis to medical care, at least in rudimentary form, dates back over 300 years, it has only been in the last 20 years that serious attention has been paid to its potential usefulness in health services applications.[10] The program administrator, as is true for all of us, is constantly faced with the need to make economic choices, given limited resources. These choices are for the most part made on the basis of a market, with the price mechanism as the regulating device. For many decisions in the public sector and some in the private sector, particularly in the health field, markets do not exist or do not function satisfactorily to produce an optimal allocation of resources.

For example, some goods, such as biomedical research, have what economists call externalities. That is, the action of one person or organization produces benefits or costs to others for which there is no compensation. In this case, private benefits or costs are not equivalent to social benefits or costs. Other frequently mentioned examples of this phenomenon are immunizations, air pollution control, and sanitation measures. For all of these, the individual or agency undertaking some action may benefit, but there are substantial additional benefits to others as well. Even in the absence of externalities, the market for a particular service may be distorted in such a way as to require some resource allocation device other than prices. For example, in the presence of complete health insurance and ready access to health services, where the price to the consumer at the time of delivery approaches zero, some other mechanism may be needed to allocate scarce resources among various possible types of service to be rendered.

Cost-benefit analysis, then, may be used as a substitute for the market. The basic principles for choice, however, are the same. That is, selection of programs or services are made on the basis of the degree to which benefits outweigh costs; theoretically, an equilibrium would be reached when the additional or marginal benefit of the last program chosen equaled its marginal cost.

Cost-benefit analysis is an extension of program evaluation in the sense that in order to measure and juxtapose the benefits and costs of various alternative programs, one must be able to empirically demonstrate that a program for which costs are incurred will in fact lead to particular benefits. Furthermore, in many cases, it is also important to know the degree to which different levels of program intervention produce different levels of benefits and the time period over which such benefits will accrue. Cost-benefit analysis is frequently undertaken by analysts who are accustomed to using secondary or existing data, and therefore inadequate attention may be paid to these relationships. The administrator needs to be alert to such problems.

The most difficult theoretical and empirical problems encountered in undertaking cost-benefit analysis are deciding what to include in measuring benefits, how to measure the benefits, and how to take into account the effect of time. The calculation of program costs is generally much more straightforward, although it may be difficult and sometimes impossible to accurately measure program costs when they arise in conjunction with the costs of some other program. Program costs are generally defined and valued in terms of anticipated dollar expenditures required to undertake the program. These expenditures are viewed as representing the "opportunity costs" of foregoing the consumption of or investment in other goods and services.

More difficult is developing a complete catalog of anticipated benefits, measuring these benefits, and placing on them a common unit of value. In order to be able to aggregate the benefits and compare them to costs, benefits are expressed in terms of dollars. The types of benefits that are appropriately included in a cost-benefit analysis are generally classified as (1) direct benefits, (2) indirect benefits, and (3) intangible benefits.

In the case of medical care, direct benefits are the savings that, as a result of the program, would accrue from avoiding the future use of services. For example, a *direct benefit* resulting from the control of hypertension would be the *avoidance of future costs* associated with the diagnosis and treatment of diseases resulting from this condition. As noted by Klarman, this is considered a direct benefit in the sense that, "it is reasonable to suppose that our economy, like others, has a vast variety of wants in the face of a totality of relatively scarce resources, so that freeing resources for other, desired objectives represents a contribution to economic welfare."[11]

Klarman goes on to describe several complications in assessing direct benefits. One that has already been mentioned in a different context is that the averted costs may arise from services that are produced jointly. Eliminating that service does not necessarily result in a reduction of costs. The second problem arises because two or more diseases may be present in the patient at the same time. Eliminating one disease may not reduce future costs to the same degree in such patients as in patients for whom it is the only disease present. Still another problem arises in estimating costs that will be experienced by survivors. It is difficult to estimate both future morbidity and future unit costs or prices.

The indirect benefits category includes benefits from avoiding premature death, disability, or some lesser impairment. The reduction of these future costs is measured in terms of avoiding loss of future earnings. There are a number of conceptual problems that the analyst must resolve. For example, cost of time lost must include the value of housewives' services. A possible solution would be to estimate them by considering the opportunity cost of a woman's foregone earnings had she been in the labor force.

Intangible benefits are those that accrue by avoiding future pain, grief, or death (per se, as opposed to the economic loss of death). Several proxies have been developed in the literature for valuing intangible benefits. No satisfactory way of placing a value on intangible benefits has been developed; however, as Klarman points out, "implicit values are being placed on human life whenever public policy decisions are made on highway design, auto safety, airport landing devices and traffic control measures, mining hazards, factory safeguards, etc."[11] More methodological work, however, needs to be done before satisfactory estimates can be applied.

Up to this point, we have not dealt explicitly with the question of benefits (and costs) as they may accrue over time. Time is important in two senses.

First, one must consider program costs and potential benefits in the context of the decision-maker's time frame. Second, the most appropriate analyses consider streams of benefits and of costs, possibly over a very long period of time. Both individuals and society have a preference for benefits sooner rather than later, with the reverse true for costs.

The first time-related consideration has to do with the dynamic nature of programs that are being compared in a cost-benefit analysis. As Williams has pointed out, "Costs are not immutable 'facts' scattered about waiting to be gathered and processed. What is a relevant cost in one context is not so in another."[12] For example, the costs each day for keeping someone on renal dialysis at home would vary depending on whether one was measuring the cost for an individual already on dialysis (with the equipment installed and the necessary experience gained) or, alternatively, the cost that would be incurred if a program were starting from scratch. These differences are incorporated in the notion of marginal costs, but the point here is that the decision-maker or analyst must think prospectively, taking into account how a new program will be integrated with the currently existing practice.

The second, and perhaps more common, way of viewing the effects of time recognizes the need to discount future benefits and costs. The most typical situation is one in which the largest costs are incurred early in a program, while the benefits may not be realized until sometime in the future. The customary method for resolving this problem is to calculate the present value of future streams of benefits and costs by using some, generally arbitrary, discount rate.

Economists disagree as to the most appropriate discount rate to use. The most commonly cited approaches to selecting a discount rate are (1) the private market interest rate (on the grounds that the money spent on investment by the government could have been used for investment in the private sector); (2) a lower rate for government projects (on the grounds that there is less risk and that government should explicitly recognize future generations' preferences); and (3) project-specific rates which reflect the risk associated with each project (recognizing that projects may vary considerably among themselves). There seems to be some agreement that a single rate is desirable, but no agreement as to what the rate should be. Rates of 7 to 10 percent seem to be widely accepted for human services programs.[11,13] It is important to note that the consequences of selecting a low discount rate versus a high discount rate can be substantial. A low rate favor programs with deferred benefits. One way of viewing it is that a high discount rate would favor programs for the older segment of the population, whereas a lower discount rate would favor programs benefiting middle-aged or younger persons.

Another difficulty that arises in cost-benefit analysis has to do with the traditional assumption that one need consider only total benefits and total costs without regard for who will be receiving the benefits or incurring the costs. While the technique assists the public decision-maker in deciding what alternative should be selected to maximize the net social benefit, it does not take into account the more practical problems of implementation—that is, the question of whether individuals or agencies can in fact be induced to undertake the program selected. This question was not a major concern in earlier applications of cost-benefit analysis, such as building dams and highways. It becomes much more consequential as projects in the human services area increasingly ". . . include not only capital costs, but also the appropriate incentives to assure that providers are willing to offer the planned services and that predicted levels of demand are realized."[14] Luft has developed a conceptual framework for extension of traditional cost-benefit analysis that takes into account the differential behavior of various subgroups affected by a proposed program, such as an ambulatory surgical center.[14]

Having accounted for, aggregated, and measured all the appropriate benefits and costs for each alternative program, one can express the relationship between benefits and costs in three different forms: (1) the internal rate of return, (2) the benefit/cost ratio, or (3) the net present value. The internal rate of return is calculated by determining that rate of interest which when applied to the future stream of differences between benefits and costs would cause the present value of the differences to be zero, or, alternatively, which would cause the present value of benefits and costs to be equal. The benefit/cost ratio is, as its name implies, the ratio of the present value of benefits to the present value of costs. The net present value is simply the arithmetic difference between the present value of the streams of benefits and costs.

Each of these ways of expressing the relationship between benefits and costs has its advantages. The internal rate of return approach has limited usefulness for social investment decisions, because it cannot be used to compare programs in different time periods, because of variations in the prevailing interest rate against which the results would be compared. The second measure, the benefit/cost ratio, has the drawback of not distinguishing between programs with similar ratios but very different absolute magnitudes. The problems inherent in the use of the internal rate of return approach and the benefit/cost ratio approach are avoided by the net present value method. While this approach is not amenable to comparison with some absolute criterion for which programs to undertake, it is useful in comparing alternative programs.[15] No matter which way the results are expressed, however, the program administrator must always bear in mind that cost-benefit analysis is inevitably based on a number of assumptions and approximations and has inherently far less precision than would appear from the rather neat display of findings that may be available.

It will be recalled that in cost-benefit analysis all the elements are expressed in dollar terms. This is a necessary convention for comparing programs with different kinds of outcomes and/or benefits. Because of the hazards of measuring and expressing benefits in dollar terms, however, an alternative method may be desirable when the outcome of various alternative programs is similar and can be expressed in the same physical units. This closely related approach is called cost-effectiveness analysis. Unlike cost-benefit analysis, cost-effectiveness analysis also requires comparable streams of benefits, since one cannot readily apply the equivalent of discount ratio to services as opposed to dollars.

Cost-effectiveness analysis is used when one might achieve the same objective (for example, a reduction in the number of days of hospitalization, the delivery of x units of mental health services, or the treatment of chronic end-stage kidney disease) by any one of several different program strategies. The analysis proceeds in a manner similar to cost-benefit analysis, with the criterion being to select that program which accomplishes the objective in the least costly manner. Obviously, the decision to try to achieve a given objective is presumed to have been made prior to undertaking the analysis of the most cost-effective modality for doing so. The greatest conceptual problem in employing cost-effectiveness analysis is that, by focusing on a single outcome that is equivalent across programmatic approaches, one is obliged to ignore other possible outcomes. If one wishes to take the latter into account, some weighting scheme or common way of expressing such outcomes must be employed, thus returning the problem to one of cost-benefit analysis.

To summarize, cost-benefit analysis is a technique that extends the results of health program evaluation into the realm of policy decision-making and formalizes the comparison of alternative programs. Benefits and costs are expressed in dollar terms on the basis of costs that are avoided or resources that are foregone by using various programmatic alternatives. Benefits are classified as being direct, indirect, or intangible, and both benefits and costs are discounted to recognize the preference for benefits that accrue in the near future and costs that occur in the distant future. The analysis is generally based on relatively crude estimates and a series of assumptions that may or may not hold in a given situation; nevertheless, cost-benefit analysis provides a useful framework for formally considering the pros and cons of various programs and a mechanism for comparing them.

In addition to the considerations discussed in this chapter, selection of an appropriate design or analytical approach will also be heavily influenced by such factors as the reliability and validity of the measures to be employed, relative ease of data collection, and the strategy for data analysis and interpretation. These issues are discussed in the following chapter.

Checklist of significant terms

Internal validity
External validity
History
Maturation
Testing
Instrumentation
Regression effect
Selection bias
Experimental attrition
Selection-maturation interaction
Selection-history interaction
Selection-treatment interaction
Testing-treatment interaction
Situational effects (reactive
   arrangements)
Multiple treatment effects

Blocking
Precision control
Frequency distribution control
Simple random sample
Stratified random sample
Cluster sample
Areal multi-stage random sample
One-shot case study
One group pretest-posttest design
Static group comparison
Pretest-posttest control group design
Solomon Four-Group Design
Posttest only control group design
Cost/benefit analysis
Cost/effectiveness analysis

Sample problem exercises

1. Drawing on readings and class discussion, evaluate Skipper, J. K., and Leonard, R. C.: Children, stress, and hospitalization: a field experiment, J. Health Soc. Behav. **9:** 275-287, 1968, according to the following issues:
   a. Diagram the type of evaluative design which you think the authors have employed. Why do you suppose they chose this design over other alternatives?
   b. What might be some important considerations other than the pros and cons of the designs themselves?
   c. Would you have used a different design—why or why not?

2. In a well-designed randomized experimental evaluation of a new health education program, the experimental group after six sessions showed a statistically significant (p < .001) increase in health knowledge over the control group on a widely used examination known for its high reliability and validity. Furthermore, the evaluators are satisfied concerning the internal and external validity of the results.
   a. Would you recommend that this program be implemented in other health agencies in the area? State *specifically* the considerations you would take into account in making your recommendation.
   b. Would your recommendation be changed at all if the results had been achieved after only three sessions?
   c. Would your recommendation be changed at all if the results had not been achieved until after eight sessions?

3. In a methadone maintenance program, heroin addicts are being provided a daily supply of methadone and given intensive vocational training. Suppose an initial evaluation based on a randomized trial shows those in the treatment program with a decline in arrests three times that of the control group. You would now like to learn more about which specific component of the program (methadone versus vocational training) is primarily responsible for the apparent success. Is it the methadone? Is it the vocational training? Or is some combination of the two producing the intended effect? You are to outline an evaluative design which addresses the issue and state why you believe your design will help provide an answer to these questions. (Assume that you can randomize subjects to whatever treatment and control group you may wish to employ.)

4. Briefly comment on the extent to which you believe the Rand Health Insurance Experiment (Newhouse, J. P.: A design for a health insurance experiment, Inquiry **11:**5-27, 1974) is subject to problems of differential attrition, refusals, and the Hawthorne effect. What suggestions does the author have for handling Hawthorne effect problems, and what do you think of his strategy?

References

1. Campbell, D. T., and Stanley, J. C.: Experimental and quasi-experimental designs for research, Skokie, Ill., 1966, Rand McNally & Company.
2. Bernstein, I. N., and others: External validity and evaluation research: a codification of problems, Sociol. Methods Res., 1975, pp. 106, 110.
3. Gilbert, J. P., and others: Assessing social innovations: an empirical base for policy. In Bennett, C. A., and Lumsdaine, A. A.,

editors: Evaluation and experiment, New York, 1975, Academic Press, Inc., p. 182.
4. Campbell, D. T., and Boruch, R. F.: Making the case for ramdomized assignment to treatments by considering the alternatives. In Bennett, C. A., and Lumsdaine, A. A., editors: Evaluation and experiment, New York, 1975, Academic Press, Inc., pp. 195-297.
5. Solomon, R. L.: An extension of control group design, Psychol. Bull. **46:**137-150, 1949.

6. Campbell, D. T.: Reforms as experiments, Am. Psychol. **24**:409-429, 1969.

7. D'Costa, A., and Sechrest, L.: Program evaluation concepts for health administrators, Washington, D.C., 1976, Department of Health, Education and Welfare, Bureau of Health Manpower.

8. Deniston, O. L., and Rosenstock, I. M.: The validity of non-experimental designs for evaluating health services, Health Serv. Rep. **88**:153-164, 1973.

9. Richardson, W. C., and others: The Seattle prepaid health care project: a comparative analysis of health services, Washington, D.C., 1976, National Center for Health Services Research.

10. Fein, R.: On measuring economic benefits of health programs. In McLachlan, G., editor: Medical history of medical care; a symposium of perspectives, London, 1971, Oxford University Press for Nuffield Provincial Hospitals Trust, pp. 179-217.

11. Klarman, H. E.: Application of cost-benefit analysis to the health services and the special case of technological innovation, Int. J. Health Serv. **4**:328-329, 331, 335, 1974.

12. Williams, A.: The cost-benefit approach, Br. Med. Bull. **30**:255, 1974.

13. Phelps, C. E.: Benefit/cost analysis of quality assurance programs. In Egdahl, R. H., editor: Quality assurance in health care, Rockville, Md., 1976, Aspen Systems Corporation, p. 291.

14. Luft, H. S.: Benefit-cost analysis and public policy implementation: from normative to positive analysis, Public Policy **24**:437-462, 1976.

15. Meenan, R. F.: The economics of biomedical research and development: an explanation and critique of cost-benefit approaches, Robert Wood Johnson Clinical Scholar Program, University of California—Stanford University, May, 1976.

Suggested readings

Bernstein, I. N., and others: External validity in evaluation research;. a codification of problems, Sociol. Methods Res., 1975, pp. 101-128.

Bunker, J. P., Barnes, B. A., and Mosteller, F.: Costs, risks, and benefits of surgery, New York, 1977, Oxford University Press, Inc.

Campbell, D. T., and Stanley, J. C.: Experimental and quasi-experimental designs for research, Skokie, Ill., 1966, Rand McNally & Company.

Cochrane, A. L.: Effectiveness and efficiency, London, 1972, Nuffield Provincial Hospitals Trust.

Gilbert, J. P., and others: Assessing social innovations: an empirical base for policy. In Bennett, C. A., and Lumsdaine, A. A., editors: Evaluation and experiment, New York, 1975, Academic Press, Inc., pp. 116-152.

Kish, L.: Survey sampling, New York, 1965, John Wiley & Sons, Inc.

Klarman, H. E.: Application of cost-benefit analysis to the health services and the special case of technological innovation, Int. J. Health Serv. **4**:325-352, 1974.

Luft, H. S.: Benefit-cost analysis and public policy implementation: from normative to positive analysis, Public Policy **24**:437-462, 1976.

Moser, C. A., and Kalton, G.: Survey methods in social investigation, ed. 2, New York, 1972, Basic Books, Inc., Publishers, pp. 61-237.

Mushkin, S. J., and Collings, F. d'A.: Economic costs of disease and injury, Public Health Rep. **74**:795-809, 1959.

Riecken, H. W., and Boruch, R. F.: Social experimentation: a method for planning and evaluating social intervention, New York, 1974, Academic Press, Inc., pp. 41-116.

Slonim, M. J.: Sampling in a nutshell, New York, 1960, Simon & Schuster, Inc.

Snedecor, G. W., and Cochran, W. G.: Statistical methods, ed. 6, Ames, 1967, Iowa State University Press, pp. 504-539.

Suchman, E.: Evaluative research: principles and practice in public service and social action programs, New York, 1967, Russell Sage Foundation, pp. 91-114.

Weiss, C. H.: Evaluation research: methods of assessing program effectiveness, Englewood Cliffs, N.J., 1972, Prentice-Hall, Inc., pp. 60-91.

CHAPTER 4

Measurement, data collection, and data analysis issues

Measurement issues—reliability and validity

Measurement is the process by which objects or events are classified or described. There are four basic levels of measurement: (1) nominal, (2) ordinal, (3) interval, and (4) ratio. *Nominal* measures include the classification of objects or events into two or more mutually exclusive classes. For example, sex is considered a nominal variable since individuals are usually classified as either male or female. Other examples include "sick or non-sick," "absent or present," "employed or not employed," and "yes or no" responses to survey questions.

Ordinal measures include classification of objects or events that differ in the *amount* of characteristics possessed, but the difference cannot be measured on a constant scale. Examples include subjective judgments of one's health status as "poor," "good," or "excellent" or one's degree of satisfaction with medical care as "very dissatisfied," "dissatisfied," "satisfied," or "very satisfied."

Interval measures include the classification of events or objects according to an instrument or scale possessing a constant interval but no true zero point or defined point of origin. With interval measures it is possible not only to say something about the *order* of observations but also about the *distance* between each observation; for example, the distance between three and four is the same as the distance between seven and eight. The important advantage of variables measured at the interval level is that they can be meaningfully added and subtracted. However, because they lack a defined point of origin, they cannot really be multiplied or divided.

Finally, *ratio* measurement includes variables in which there is not only a constant interval between observation points but also a true zero point or defined point of origin on the scale. As such, it becomes possible to multiply and divide numbers meaningfully. Examples of ratio measures include family size, family income, number of days to get a doctor's appointment, travel time to the doctor's office, and so on.

Regardless of the level of measurement, issues of reliability and validity emerge. This was referred to in Chapter 3 as instrumentation bias, which is a potential threat to internal validity. Although many of the threats to internal validity, such as history and maturation, may be guarded against through appropriate choice of design, instrumentation error can be strictly guarded against only by selection of reliable and valid measures. If doubt exists regarding the reliability and validity of individual measures, then both the internal validity and external validity of the evaluation results must be questioned. The need for reliable and valid measures is particularly important if program effects are expected to be small and sample sizes are small. This section discusses basic issues related to the reliability and validity of individual measures and provides several different methods for assessing each.

Definitions

Reliability may be defined as the extent to which the *same measure* gives the same results on *repeated applications*. The concern is with assessing chance or *random error*. For example, a survey designed to measure patient satisfaction might be given to the same respondents in both the morning and the afternoon. If the survey is to be a reliable measure of patient satisfaction, there must be a high degree of correlation between the two administrations (for example, .75 or higher). Failure to obtain a high degree of correlation may be due to inconsistencies in the reports of those individuals being studied, inconsistencies in the judgments of raters or observers, differences in the situation in which data are collected, subtle changes in the measuring instrument itself, or errors in data processing.

Validity refers to the extent to which a measure really measures what it *purports to measure.* Its concern is with *systematic error*—that is, changes that are a part of the natural variation in the phenomenon under study. For example, does the number of annual disability days really measure a person's health status? In other words, is number of disability days a *valid* measure of health status? Is the concept "health status" captured by or truly reflected in the measure "annual bed disability days?" Such an assessment usually involves comparing *two different measures* of some variable or phenomenon, unlike reliability which always involves assessing the same measure. Potential sources of invalidity include those mentioned earlier for reliability (subject variability, observer variability, and so on) plus errors resulting from biased sampling, poor administration of data collection, and deficiencies in analysis of particular measures.

Reliability is a necessary, but not sufficient, condition for validity. It is not possible to have a valid measure that is not also reliable; however, it is possible to have a measure that is reliable but not necessarily valid. For example, age-adjusted blood pressure could not be considered a valid outcome measure of quality of care for hypertensive patients if their blood pressures were not reliably measured. If a measure is not reliable, one can say little regarding its potential validity. On the other hand, a variable may be reliably measured but not be a valid measure of a particular concept. For example, a person's height may be measured reliably but would certainly not be considered a valid measure of a person's health status. Or, to cite a more realistic example, days absent from school may be measured reliably but may not at all be a valid measure of a child's health status. Some absenteeism may be due to family vacations, family trips, observance of ethnic or religious holidays, and other factors not related to childhood illness. In sum, a valid measure must by definition be reliable, but a reliable measure will not not necessarily be a valid measure.

Types and methods of assessing reliability

Data may be collected by observing people's behavior or by tests, questionnaires, and related survey methodologies. For each of these general categories of measurement, reliability may be assessed at the *same point in time* or *at different points in time*. For each of these and for each of the different ways of collecting data, a number of different methods are available for assessing reliability. These are summarized in Table 6 and discussed here.

When the measurement method involves observers, reliability may be assessed at the same point in time by computing inter-rater or inter-observer reliability coefficients (see cell A in Table 6). This simply involves correlating the judgments and ratings made by the different observers at the same point in time. This is sometimes referred to as "objectivity reliability." For example, one could assemble ten physician experts to rate the importance of various diagnostic items in providing high-quality care for diabetic patients. The reliability of their judgments could then be assessed by correlating their ratings (that is, inter-rater correlations). The higher the average inter-rater correlation, the more reliable the measure. It is also possible to assess the reliability of individual rater's judgments over time. That is, one might be interested in the extent to which individual physician's ratings are consistent from one time period to the next. Thus, physicians might be asked to make their ratings twice, perhaps several days apart. This involves correlating the ratings made by the same physician in response to the same item at different points in time. Such an intra-rater or intra-observer reliability coefficient may be termed a measure of "precision reliability" (see cell B in Table 6).

Where the measurement method involves tests or questionnaire items, reliability may be assessed at the same point in time by computing split-half re-

Table 6. Summary of reliability assessment methods

Measurement method	Time interval	
	Same point in time	*Different points in time*
Observers/raters	Inter-rater or inter-observer reliability; correlate judgments made by different observers at same point in time "Objectivity reliability" (A)	Intra-rater and intra-observer reliability; correlate judgments made by the same person at two different points in time "Precision reliability" (B)
Tests, question-naires, surveys	Split-half reliability; short-form vs. long form; internal consistency reliability "Congruence reliability" (C)	"Test-retest reliability" (D)

liability coefficients, by correlating responses to short forms versus long forms of questionnaires, and by a variety of internal consistency checks in which basically identical questions are worded somewhat differently (see cell C in Table 6). These methods may be thought of as examples of "congruence reliability." Split-half reliability assessments are particularly appropriate for health knowledge questionnaires. For a questionnaire with thirty statements, one would randomly split them into two halves of fifteen questions each and correlate the two halves. If the questionnaire is reliable, one should expect no more true or false, or positive or negative, answers on one half than on the other. Individuals' scores on one half should be similar to their scores on the other half. This will be reflected in a high correlation between the two halves of the test. Various formulas are available for computing split-half reliability coefficients.[1]

In some cases it may be possible to administer a long *and* a short version of a questionnaire. One can then assess the extent to which responses to identical questions are similar in the two versions. This is frequently done in pretesting a study instrument to see if it is possible to use a shorter version that will require less time of the respondent. If the shorter version yields similar results, then the evaluator can save time and money by using it. It is also possible to build internal consistency checks into the questionnaire by slightly altering the wording of basically identical questions. For example, in a health knowledge test the following questions might appear:

1. Can extreme shortness of breath be a sign of heart disease? (yes or no)
2. Can one possible indicator of heart disease be extreme difficulty in breathing? (yes or no)

If the questionnaire is reliable, one expects respondents to give the same answer each time. That is, if they answer yes (or no) to the first question, they should also answer yes (or no) to the second. It is, of course, important in designing such questions that they not be placed in immediate proximity to each other but be distributed at wide intervals throughout the questionnaire.

When tests or questionnaires are the method of measurement, it is also possible to assess reliability at different points in time through the use of test-retest correlations (see cell D in Table 6). For example, the health knowledge examination could be administered at two different points in time, perhaps 1 week apart. One would then compute a test-retest correlation of the two test administrations. A key issue involves selecting the time interval for the retest. If too short a period is selected, reliability may be overestimated because respondents may simply remember how they answered the first time and repeat the same response. On the other hand, if too long a period is used then *genuine changes* may have occurred in the respondent's level of health knowledge. In such cases, the retest is not a reliability check on the original test. Rather, the issue becomes one of *validity* in terms of how quickly the phenomenon under question (in this case, health knowledge) is supposed to change. The same issue applies to intra-observer reliability, previously discussed. In the case of a health knowledge examination, a 1- to 2-week interval would seem appropriate since it is unlikely that respondents could recall many of their answers after 1 or 2 weeks and, at the same time, it is unlikely that their actual level of health knowledge (in the absence of a particular program intervention or extremely salient event) will have genuinely changed.

Factors to consider

A particular method of assessing reliability will depend on the *measure* being used, the *phenomenon* under study, *cost and logistics, time,* and the extent to which *previous assessments* of reliability have been made. If *people* (either observers or raters) are being used as the measuring instrument, then, obviously, inter- or intra-reliability is involved. If *tests or questionnaires* are involved, then split-half, internal consistency, and test-retest methods may be used. If the phenomenon under study is expected to change quickly, then a measure of reliability "at the same point in time" (for example, inter-rater in the case of raters or split-half in the case of tests or questionnaires) is the method of choice. The costs and logistics of program operation will also affect methods of assessing reliability. In particular, attempting to assess reliability at two different points in time may run into cost and logistical problems. The method of reliability selected will also be a function of the *amount of time available* before the program is to begin. The greater the length of time available, the easier it is to conduct intra-observer and test-retest reliability assessments.

Finally, the reliability of a particular measure may already be known, based on *previous calculations.* In such cases, the evaluators may not need to assess a particular measure's reliability or may need a less rigorous assessment than would otherwise be true. This depends on the extent to which the measure was previously used in an evaluation *similar* to the one under study. In cases where the reliability of a particular measure has been determined in evaluations quite *different* from the one of immediate concern, the measure's reliability should be assessed anew within the context of the present program.

Types and methods for assessing validity

There are five major types of validity assessment: *face* validity, *content* validity, *concurrent* validity, *predictive* validity, and *construct* validity. It is important to note that all include some form of judgment or consensus. *Face* validity involves common acceptance by all concerned that a particular measure indeed measures what it purports to measure. It involves the principle of *res ipsa loquitor* (the thing speaks for itself). For example, almost everyone would agree that people dying of cancer are in poor physical health.

Content validity concerns the extent to which a measure or test represents a reasonable sample of the total behaviors or attributes that comprise the variable of interest. It is normally determined by soliciting the agreement of relevant judges. For example, if medical experts working independently developed measures of the quality of care for treatment of diabetes that yielded equivalent results, one would say that the measures exhibited content validity. In contrast, if the measures yielded widely different results, one would question their content validity.

Concurrent (or convergent) validity involves the correlation of one measure with another at the *same point in time.* It is particularly appropriate when a single good measure is not available. If two different measures of the same phenomenon are highly correlated, one can have greater confidence that the phenomenon under study is being validly measured. For example, if both laboratory and x-ray tests are in agreement, a physician may have more confidence in the validity of a particular diagnosis. Of, if a patient's self-report of poor health status correlates highly with the results of a clinical examination, one has greater confidence in the validity of self-report data as a valid measure of health status.

Predictive validity concerns the extent to which a current measure is predictive of some future event. For example, if on the basis of a health knowledge test it is possible to predict an individual's future response to symptoms, then the health knowledge test is said to have predictive validity. It is important to note that both concurrent validity and predictive validity are forms of *criterion validity*. Criterion validity involves comparing one measure with another measure that is felt in some way to be "more valid." The more valid measure constitutes the *criterion* against which the other measure is assessed. In the case of concurrent validity, one measure is assessed against a criterion measure at the same point in time, while in predictive validity the concern is with different measures at different points in time. In the case of predictive validity, the future event is always adopted as the criterion ("most valid") measure. But in the case of concurrent validity, a choice needs to be made between the two measures. The general rule is to select as the criterion that measure which on the basis of face or content validity appears to be more closely related to the phenomenon of interest. Thus, in the earlier example of a patient's self-report of health status and a clinical examination, the latter might be considered the criterion measure against which patient self-reports are to be assessed.

Construct validity involves situations in which there is no reasonable criterion variable and no common acceptance regarding content validity. The concern is with trying to measure some attribute or phenomenon that is not well-defined. A *construct* is essentially a postulated attribute for people or events that is assumed to be reflected in a particular measure. For example, intelligence is what intelligence tests measure, or mental health is what psychiatrists and psychologists say it is.

The selection of a particular method of assessing validity will depend on many of the factors previously discussed for reliability (phenomenon involved, cost, logistics, time, and so on). In some cases, face validity or content validity will be sufficient. For example, it is commonly accepted that cost per standardized unit of output is one valid measure of program efficiency. In other cases, previous validity assessments of a particular measure may have been made. But in many cases evaluators will be required to assess the validity of particular measures of key variables. This is particularly true with newer measures and with variables that are ill-defined. In such cases, a useful method of both reliability and validity assessment involves application of the multi-trait, multi-method matrix.[2]

Multi-trait, multi-method matrix

The multi-trait, multi-method matrix was originally developed by educational psychologists interested in assessing the validity of different tests to measure intelligence and educational achievement. The term "trait" refers to a specific attribute to be measured, for example, patient satisfaction, physical health, or level of health knowledge. The term "method" refers to a specific means or procedure of measuring various traits or attributes. Examples include self-administered questionnaires, personal interview, or direct observation. The basic idea is to compare *different* methods of measuring the *same* trait, the *same* method of measuring *different* traits, and *different* methods of measuring *different* traits. The purpose of such comparisons is best illustrated by the example shown in Fig. 8.

In this figure, there are three different traits or concepts being measured, namely, physical health status (PH), mental health status (MH), and extroversion (EXT). There are also three different methods of measurement, namely, a survey questionnaire (SQ), a physical dysfunction index (PDI), and clinical examination (CE). The numbers in parentheses indicate the reliability coefficients for each measure, for example, based on split-half or test-retest reliabilities. (See Note 1 of Fig. 8.) If these were not sufficiently high, there would be no need to examine the figure any further, since we know from previous discussion that unreliable measures cannot be valid. The numbers in parentheses in Fig. 8, however, indicate a high degree of reliability; thus, the main concern is with determining the validity of the measures.

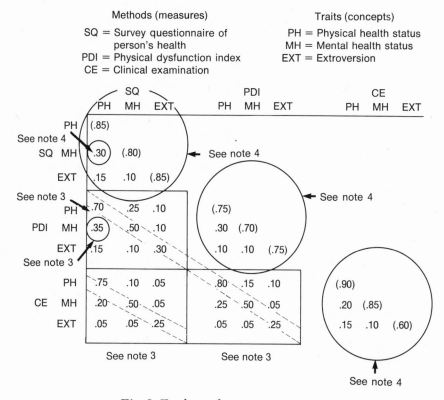

Fig. 8. For legend see opposite page.

Fig. 8. Multi-trait, multi-method matrix example.

1. The numbers in parentheses indicate the reliability coefficients, for example, (.85).
2. The numbers within the dashed lines (⟍⟍) indicate the *convergent validity* coefficients, that is, the extent to which *two different methods (measures)* of measuring the *same concept* are correlated with each other. In order to have some evidence of convergent validity, these coefficients should at least be significantly different from zero. This, of course, will depend upon the size of the sample upon which the data are based.
3. The numbers within the square boxes (except for the convergent validity coefficients within the dashed lines) indicate the correlation between *two different concepts* using *two different measures*. For example, in the first square box, we see that the correlation between physical health and mental health, using the Survey Questionnaire (SQ) to measure physical health and the Physical Dysfunction Index (PDI) to measure mental health, is .35 (the circled number). When we compare these "off diagonal" coefficients with those within the diagonal (within the dashed lines) we hope to find that those within the diagonal are higher than those off the diagonal, for purposes of giving some evidence of discriminant validity. This is because the diagonal coefficients (the convergent validity coefficients) indicate the correlation between two different measures of the *same concept*, while the other coefficients indicate the correlation between different measures of *different concepts*. If we found these latter coefficients to be nearly as high as the former we would not be at all sure of whether we were measuring physical health or mental health. Depending on the sample size, a rough rule of thumb is that the convergent validity coefficients within the dashed lines should be approximately $1\frac{1}{2}$ to 2 times the magnitude of the other coefficients within the box.
4. The numbers within the large circles (except for the reliability measures which are in parentheses) indicate the correlation between *two different concepts* using *the same method*. Thus, in the first circle we see that the correlation between physical health and mental health, using the Survey Questionnaire as the measure, is .30 (the circled number). If we wanted to know whether we were validly measuring physical health status, we would certainly hope that the correlation between physical health and mental health is not very high—certainly, at least, not as high as our two independent measures of physical health (SQ and PDI) which, in this case, are shown to be correlated at .70 (see the first number in the first validity diagonal). If the correlation between physical health and mental health were high (say, close to .70) we really would not know whether we were measuring physical health or mental health status! Thus, for purposes of discriminant validity, we hope that the convergent validity coefficients within the dashed lines are larger in magnitude than the corresponding coefficients in the columns and rows of the large circles.
5. In addition to the above, if we can show that the *pattern* of correlations within the large circles and square boxes are *generally the same*, we have some further evidence of discriminant validity. For example, given the data outlined above, we see that the correlations between physical health and mental health are *always higher* than those between physical health and extroversion, and mental health and extroversion. We also see that the correlations between physical health and extroversion are always as high as or higher than those between mental health and extroversion.

The key advantage of the multi-trait, multi-method matrix is that it provides data on both *convergent* (concurrent) and *discriminant* validity. Convergent validity has been previously discussed (pp. 78–79) and involves the extent to which two different measures of the same attribute are correlated. The correlation should be significantly different from zero in the statistical sense (that is, "probably" have not occurred by chance where the probability is known). The higher the correlation, the greater the convergent validity of the attribute being measured. In Fig. 8, convergent validity coefficients are indicated by the numbers within the dashed diagonal lines. (See Note 2 of Fig. 8.) For example, the correlation between the SQ and PDI measures of physical health is .70. The correlation between the SQ and PDI measures of mental health is .50, and so on. Given a sufficiently large sample size (for example, 100 individuals), these correlations would be statistically significant.

But, in addition to evidence of convergent validity, the multi-trait, multi-method approach requires that a particular method of measurement should *not* be highly correlated with some other method of measurement from which it is *intended to differ*. This is referred to as *discriminant validity* and represents a much more stringent test of the validity of a particular measure. It is one thing to show that two different measures of the same phenomenon are highly correlated but quite another to show that neither of these measures is highly correlated with a third measure for which no correlation is expected. If high correlations were obtained, then one must doubt the overall validity of the first two measures even though they may have exhibited convergent validity. The three requirements for discriminant validity are described below.

The first requirement is that the convergent validity correlations lying within the diagonal dashed lines *should be higher than the values lying in their respective columns and rows involving different measures of different traits*. (See Note 3 of Fig. 8.) For example, in Fig. 8 it is seen that .70, representing the correlation between SQ and PDI in measuring physical health (two different methods of measuring the same trait), is higher than .35 (in the circle), which is the correlation between the SQ measure of physical health and the PDI measure of mental health (two different measures of two different traits). It can also be seen that .70 is higher than all the other off-diagonal correlations in that square.

The second requirement for discriminant validity is that the correlation between two different methods of measuring the same trait (that is, the convergent validity correlations) should be greater than the correlation between two different traits using the *same* method. (See Note 4 of Fig. 8.) In Fig. 8 it is seen that .70, which is the correlation of the SQ and PDI measures of physical health (the convergent validity correlations representing two different measures of the same trait), is higher than .30 (in the circle), which is the correlation *between* the SQ measure of mental health and the SQ measure of physical health (the correlation of two different traits measured by the *same* method). As can be seen, .70 is also higher than the other non-parenthesis correlations in the large circles.

The third, but somewhat less important, requirement for discriminant validity is that the same general pattern of correlations among traits should be observed in all of the triangles. (See Note 5 of Fig. 8.) For example, in Fig. 8 it is seen that the correlations between physical health (PH) and mental health (MH) are always higher than those between physical health (PH) and extroversion (EXT), or between mental health (MH) and extroversion (EXT). Also, the correlations between physical health (PH) and extroversion (EXT) are either higher or at least of the same magnitude as those between mental health (MH) and extroversion (EXT).

Two guidelines are useful in setting up a multi-trait, multi-method assessment of validity. First, care should be taken that measurement methods are selected that differ sufficiently so that a high correlation between two measures cannot occur because of the inherent similarity of the two measurement methods. This might occur, for example, if two almost identical questionnaires are used. In Fig. 8, assume that the SQ, PDI, and CE measures are sufficiently different to meet this guideline. Second, select at least one trait or attribute that is believed to be independent of the other two. In the case of Fig. 8, inclusion of the trait "extroversion" meets this guideline. In other words, if the goal is to assess the validity of a particular measure—for example, physical health—we might expect some correlation between physical health and mental health but should certainly not expect a very strong correlation with extroversion. If a strong correlation with extroversion were obtained, one would be forced to question seriously the validity of the measure of physical health. If our assumed measure of physical health is so highly correlated with extroversion, how do we know we are not measuring extroversion rather than physical health status? While one trait should be selected that is believed to be "different" from the other traits, the greater the extent to which this trait is *somewhat conceptually related* to the other traits, the stronger is the test of discriminant validity. "Conceptually related" means that the trait selected is not totally unrelated to the basic meaning of the other traits. For example, if the goal were to determine the discriminant validity of a math examination, a strong test would include verbal scores and overall IQ (all three being traits generally considered under the broad rubric of "intelligence") rather than such traits as introspection or attitudes toward authority. While the multi-trait, multi-method matrix provides a rigorous assessment of measurement validity, the time, effort, and cost associated with its use preclude actual implementation in many evaluations. Nevertheless, its concepts and rationale provide evaluators, providers, program administrators, and planners with a clear understanding of measurement validity issues. When opportunities arise, and in particular when new measures of little-understood concepts are being used, serious consideration should be given to using multiple measures and multiple concepts and assessing their convergent and discriminant validity.

Summary of reliability and validity issues

Table 7 summarizes the difference and relationship between reliability and validity. It should be noted that the reliability and validity issues raised in this chapter apply to *all* measures being used in a potential program evaluation. This is true regardless of whether the concern is with measuring program effort, performance, performance relative to need, efficiency, or process. It is

Table 7. Summary of reliability and validity issues

Characteristics	Reliability	Validity
1. Definition	Is concerned with the degree to which the same measure yields consistent results upon repeated application	Is concerned with the degree to which a particular measure reflects what it is supposed to measure
2. Nature of error measured	Is concerned with chance or random error	Is concerned with systematic error—i.e., natural variation in the phenomenon under study
3. Relationship	Reliability is necessary for validity	Validity is not necessary for reliability
4. Types	Inter-rater, intra-rater, split-half, test-retest	Face, content, concurrent (convergent), predictive, construct
5. Sources of error	Subjects, observers, situations, instruments, processing	Same as for reliability plus errors due to sampling, data collection, administration, and analysis
6. Level of significance necessary	Depends on the degree of validity required; the greater the degree of validity required, the greater the need for higher reliability coefficients	If the program results are to be used for internal improvement only, one might be willing to accept somewhat lower validity coefficients; in contrast, if the program is to be generalized to other settings and be given wide exposure, more stringent (higher) validity coefficients are likely to be used

also true regardless of whether the unit of analysis is program clients, effect on the agency itself, effect on large systems, or effect on the public at large.

Data collection—issues and strategies

A variety of methods for collecting data is available. The most "appropriate" method(s) for a given case will depend on the nature of the program being evaluated (objectives, specification of program components, and so on), the variables to be measured, the evaluation design being employed, and the cost and time involved. For evaluation of an ongoing program, it may be possible to reconstruct "baseline" data by making use of existing program resources. But for a new program, one may need to collect original data and possibly institute an entire data collection and monitoring system from start. When the objectives involved can be readily measured in quantifiable terms, existing data bases and existing "social indicators" may be used. But when the objectives are more concerned with measuring changes in participants' attitudes or beliefs, interviews or survey questionnaires become the method of choice. If time is of the essence and funds are in short supply, then by necessity primary reliance will have to be placed on existing data. Without such constraints, consideration can be given to the appropriateness of interviews, questionnaires, and related survey methodologies.

As mentioned, the two primary means of data collection are using *existing (precollected) data* and using *original data collection*. The advantages and disadvantages of each of these are discussed in the following paragraphs.

Precollected data

Two principal types of precollected data are *archival records* and an agency's *administrative records*.[3] Archival records refer to existing historical data that may be available from a number of sources other than the organization whose program is being evaluated. Examples in the health field include the various statistical services of the National Center for Health Statistics, the morbidity and mortality reports of the Center for Disease Control, the Professional Activities Study and Medical Audit Program (PAS-MAP) of the Commission on Professional and Hospital Activities, and the Hospital Administrative Services (HAS) Program of the American Hospital Association. Administrative records of the program itself might include financial, utilization, personnel, and associated data related to the program's operation. It is frequently the case that data collected on the experimental program itself will come from the organization involved with the program while, assuming a control or comparison group in the evaluation design, data collected on other groups in the evaluation will come not only directly from them but from archival sources as well.

A third form of precollected data involves *unobtrusive* measures.[4] Unobtrusive measures may be considered "precollected" in the sense that evaluators may observe the effect of previous events or processes without asking people directly or indirectly for information. For example, a program intended to eliminate paper wastage on working units might be evaluated by observing and recording the volume of paper in wastepaper baskets. A program designed to increase exchange of information between two health delivery organizations might be assessed with a count of the number of calls (through the telephone switchboard) made by both organizations to each other. Since a major problem of unobtrusive measures is their appropriateness, primary emphasis here is given to other data sources based on existing activities or administrative records.

Advantages. The primary advantage of precollected data, both archival and administrative records, is its *low cost* relative to other forms of data collection. While such data frequently cannot be used in the forms in which they exist, the cost of transforming them to suit the purpose of the evaluation is usually less than having to collect the same data from scratch.

The second major advantage of precollected data is that they can frequently be used as "baseline" or "pretest" measures in before/after evaluation designs. They are particularly useful with time series designs. Furthermore, in the case of archival records, they frequently affect *comparability* across the different organizations or programs involved in the research.[3] This is particularly true of data collected by federal agencies on a required basis (such as morbidity and mortality reports) and less true of private organizations and associations (such as PAS-MAP) where clients subscribe on a voluntary basis.

Disadvantages. The principal disadvantages of precollected data are its potential *incompleteness, inaccuracy,* and *inappropriateness.* Densen, commenting on the potential to evaluate utilization and cost savings in a prepaid group practice, notes:

> Both the decision not to include the utilization of physician's services on the tape and the decision to suspend the 5 percent sample were presumably taken for reasons of economy. But as a result, the task of rendering account is made inordinately difficult and may in the long run increase instead of decrease costs. The first decision affects the ability to determine the utilization factors which determine expenditures; the second makes it very difficult, except through very special and costly procedures, to obtain appropriate comparison populations to match with study populations. Both decisions decrease management's flexibility to assess the program. One could wish for more effective communication between the policy makers and epidemiologists when these decisions are being considered.[5]

But even data sources that are complete and accurate may be *inappropriate* as a measure of a particular variable. For example, an agency's records of broken appointments may be complete and accurate but may not be at all an appropriate (in the sense of "valid") measure of client satisfaction. Failure to keep appointments may reflect a belief that the services are not necessary or that there are problems with child care, transportation, and so on, rather than dissatisfaction with the agency's services.

In addition to the problems of incompleteness, inaccuracy, and inappropriateness, administrative records have the further limitation of frequently not being comparable across sites. Thus, it is not often possible to compare one program's performance with another because the relevant variables involved have been measured in different ways with incomparable data sets. A major thrust of federal as well as private association evaluation efforts in recent years has been to standardize information reporting systems for the purpose of being able to draw some basic comparisons. A notable example is the Uniform Hospital Discharge Data Set developed by the Department of Health, Education and Welfare in conjunction with the American Hospital Association.[6]

Finally, it is also necessary to make sure that the way in which administrative data has been collected does not change during the course of the evaluation. Changes in the definition of terms or the kinds of data being collected can invalidate an evaluation since the postexperimental data may not be comparable with the pre-experimental program data.

In sum, many precollected data are particularly useful (1) in cases where program objectives can easily be measured with available data, (2) as a source of baseline measures in before/after evaluation designs, and (3) in single group and multiple group time-series analyses. Existing data can also be a useful source of information for cost-benefit and cost-effectiveness analyses. Finally, there exist cases in which precollected data is the only practical alternative available. The evaluator must assess the accuracy, reliability, and validity of the data and decide whether it is "good enough" to go forward with the evaluation. In cases where the impact of the program is expected to be large, less than optimal data may be sufficient to proceed ahead. Errors in such data will affect the relative magnitude of program impact but not the validity of the impact itself. In contrast, in situations where there is considerable doubt about a particular program's impact, it is extremely dangerous to rely on data whose accuracy, reliability, or validity may be questioned. Reliance on such data may lead to the wrong conclusion regarding program impact. In these cases it might be best to forego an impact evaluation altogether and instead develop a process-oriented monitoring evaluation that might provide more reliable and valid data for future impact evaluations.

Original data collection

The development of routine *ongoing* data collection systems represents one form of original data collection. Their importance, particularly for prospective evaluations, needs to be recognized. A good example is the data required for concurrent reviewing of the quality of hospital care being developed by the Professional Standards Review Organizations (PSROs) in conjunction with individual hospital medical staffs. However, even the best designed ongoing data collection systems are limited by some of the disadvantages cited earlier in regard to precollected data. It is difficult to anticipate evaluative needs in advance and frequently not as easy, in fact, to adapt existing data collection systems to new developments as is possible in theory. In brief, many evaluations will require data beyond that already available or currently being obtained. This most frequently takes the form of questionnaires.

Questionnaires may be used in a personal interview format, in a telephone interview, or may be self-administered (filled in by the respondent). In addition, the questions asked may be either open-ended or closed-ended. Open-ended questions allow the respondent to reply in any way desired. The following is an example: "How do you feel about the quality of care provided by nurse practitioners?" To the extent possible, the interviewer then records verbatim the respondent's reply. In closed-ended questions, the response categories are determined in advance, and the respondent indicates a particular choice to the interviewer (or circles a particular number in the case of a self-administered questionnaire). The following is an example:

The quality of care provided by nurse practitioners is:

Excellent	1
Good	2
Fair	3
Poor	4

Interview questionnaires—advantages and disadvantages. Questionnaires are particularly useful in measuring individual attitudes and opinions. They are generally less useful in obtaining factual information. The primary advantage of open-ended questionnaires is that they allow for a full range of opinion to be expressed. With the appropriate use of probing (by asking follow-up questions, such as, "What else?"), it is possible to obtain a rich and detailed base of information on various issues. The disadvantages of open-ended questions are the amount of time involved and the lack of comparability in responses that creates problems in coding data and data processing. These disadvantages are the exact advantages of closed-ended or "structured" questionnaires. They generally require less time to complete, are associated with increased comparability of response (but do not always guarantee comparability), and are easier to process. Their primary disadvantage is that they may unnecessarily force respondents into selecting particular categories. In general, when much is known about the range of valid responses to a particular question, it is safe to develop a closed-ended question with predetermined response categories. In contrast, when little is known about an issue, it is usually preferable to use an open-ended question. Open-ended questions are particularly useful in process evaluation and implementation assessments. When adequate time and funds are available, it is possible to use an open-ended questionnaire in a pretest or pilot study and from respondent replies develop a set of predetermined responses to be used in a closed-ended questionnaire during the actual study itself. Some questionnaires will employ both approaches to a particular issue. An open-ended question will be asked first so that the respondent can elaborate in some depth and then this will be followed by a closed-ended question to force the respondent to state a summary judgment of the issue in question.

   Self-administered questionnaires—advantages and disadvantages. Self-administered questionnaires usually take less time than interviews, are less costly, and avoid possible interviewer bias. The latter refers to situations in which interviewers may influence responses by the manner in which questions are asked. Bias may be introduced through verbal (tone of voice) or nonverbal (gestures) means. In terms of disadvantages, while self-administered questionnaires can be open-ended, the richness of detail gained by being able to ask probing follow-up questions is largely lost, instructions or questions cannot be further clarified, and typically, but not always, completion rates are lower. Self-administered questionnaires are particularly appropriate if the information to be obtained is well-structured, a large number of respondents is involved, and funds are limited.

   Telephone interviews—advantages and disadvantages. Telephone interviews are becoming increasingly useful. They offer many of the advantages of direct interviews and self-administered questionnaires without the associated disadvantages. They are often cheaper than direct interviews, although they may not be as cheap as mailed self-administered questionnaires, and may not be much cheaper than direct interviews when dealing with probability samples. Instructions and questions can be clarified and explained over the telephone, and nonverbal bias can be eliminated. The primary disadvantages of telephone interviews are that respondents may not have enough time to reflect properly on each question and there is greater risk that the interview will be broken off before completion. A useful strategy is to use telephone interviews in combination with sending an advance questionnaire. This enables the respondent to refer to the questionnaire as the questions are being asked.

It also alerts the respondent in advance to the general length and context of the interview so that a psychological set is created prior to the phone call.

Summary of data collection strategies

The advantages and disadvantages of each major data collection method are summarized in Table 8. None has been treated in any depth in this section since there are several good texts available that do provide such coverage (see Suggested Readings). However, several general points need to be highlighted.

First, it is usually good strategy to begin by closely examining the availability and quality of existing data. Only if existing data are not readily available, or not of the quality or content appropriate to the evaluation, should consideration be given to collecting original data. Second, if original data collection is required, a thorough search for and analysis of existing measures should be made before one attempts to design new measures from scratch. Particular emphasis should be given to reports of the reliability and validity of existing measures and the extent to which the measure has been used in situations similar to the evaluation about to be undertaken. Several monographs and books are available summarizing current social science and health services measures.[7-14] Consulting such sources may not only save evaluators much time but also help to ensure comparability of measures across different program evaluation settings, thus contributing to the development of cumulative knowledge for purposes of program planning and policy analysis.

In some cases, however, existing measures will be inappropriate for a particular program evaluation. In such cases evaluators will indeed need to develop from scratch their own questions and measuring instruments. Time and funds permitting, it is extremely important that such measures be checked for reliability and validity (see previous section) and thoroughly pretested before being used in the actual evaluation. If this is not possible, a difficult decision must be made regarding whether to proceed with the evaluation. Certainly, any results obtained will need to be qualified in the face of measures of unknown reliability or validity. If the stakes are high and/or the program impact is expected to be small, it may be wiser to forego the formal evaluation in the face of measures of unknown reliability or validity. If the program is less salient and program impacts are expected to be large, it may make sense to continue the evaluation even though it is not possible to test the reliability and validity of the measures being used. This may be particularly true if the measures contain considerable face validity so they at least appear plausible to users of the evaluation report.

While the preceding outlines a general approach to be taken for data collection, it is particularly important to highlight the problem of *memory recall* with survey questionnaires. The less salient the event and the longer the time period of recall involved, the less accurate will be the response. Annual physician visits, for example, are typically underreported. The more salient the event (such as hospitalization) and the shorter the period of recall involved (for example, 2 weeks), the more accurate the reporting. Sensitive information is also less likely to be reported accurately. Table 9 shows the re-

Table 8. Summary of advantages and disadvantages of precollected and original data collection methods

Method	Advantages	Disadvantages	Best use
A. Precollected			
1. Archival, e.g., NHS, PAS-MAP	1. Less expensive 2. Often offers longitudinal data on experimental and control groups	May be incomplete, inaccurate, inappropriate (e.g., trying to measure satisfaction by broken appointment rates)	Time series analysis and designs; trying to buttress after-the-fact evaluations
2. Administrative records, e.g., hospital, clinic, agency	1. Less expensive 2. May also offer before/after measures	1. May not be comparable with comparison groups or other sites 2. Need to make sure the record system was not changed during the experimental period 3. Incomplete 4. Inaccurate 5. Inappropriate	Time series, cost-benefit, cost-effectiveness analyses; when other sources are not available
B. Original			
1. Interview questionnaires a. Structured, closed-ended	1. Relevance to issue at hand 2. Easier processing 3. Comparability	1. May unnecessarily force respondents into categories 2. Expensive	When you have an idea of the range of valid responses
b. Open-ended	1. Richness 2. Allows full range of opinion	1. Takes time 2. Problems of analysis 3. Noncomparability 4. Expensive	When little is known about a topic and for process evaluations and implementation assessments
2. Self-administered questionnaires, tests, and diaries	1. Usually takes less time 2. Less costly 3. Avoids interviewer bias	1. Lose the richness of probing 2. Instruction cannot be further explained 3. Completion rates typically lower	Small amounts of fairly well structured information to be obtained; particularly where large numbers of people are involved
3. Telephone interviewing	1. Less expensive 2. Can explain 3. Avoids nonverbal bias existent in a face-to-face interview	1. Respondents may not have time to reflect properly 2. Easier for respondent to "break off" the interview	In combination with sending a questionnaire in advance

Table 9. Hypothetical willingness to report medical conditions in relation to percentage of cases actually reported*

Condition	Percent willing to report (students)	Percent valid reports in household survey
Asthma	84	71
Heart disease	58	60
Hernia	55	54
Malignant neoplasm	31	33
Mental disease	19	25
Genitourinary disease	14	22

*From Cobb, S., and Cannell, C. F.: Some thoughts about interview data, Int. Epidemiol. Assoc. Bull. **13**:43-54, 1966.

sults of a study comparing the extent to which college students would be willing to report the existence of several chronic diseases with the actual percentage of valid reports made by respondents in a separate household survey.[15] As can be seen, the more socially sensitive the disease category, the less valid the response.

Finally, it should be noted that most program evaluations will require a combination of precollected and original data collection. Other than proceeding from existing data to existing measures for original data collection to developing new measures for original data collection, no guidelines or rules-of-thumb are available for how such data might be combined. Such decisions will challenge the creativity of the evaluator and will act as a useful reminder that the techniques and methodologies learned in graduate school cannot be automatically or routinely applied in practice. By definition, each situation will be somewhat different and the evaluator needs to combine a working knowledge of the particular situational circumstances with the principles and techniques of evaluation research to arrive at a practical solution.

Data analysis issues

Let us assume that the evaluator has been able to obtain a clear understanding of specific program objectives stated in measurable terms. He has also obtained a clear understanding of the nature of the program and its various subcomponents. He has chosen an evaluative design that permits the strongest inferences possible, given the ethical, political, and administrative constraints of the situation. He has carefully assessed the reliability and validity of specific measures and has carefully considered alternative strategies for collecting the data. Thus, the evaluator has on hand a more or less reliable and more or less valid set of data that should indicate something about the extent to which the program in question is meeting its objectives. The next issue to be addressed concerns how the data should be analyzed.

It is not the intention here to teach future evaluators, providers, program administrators, or planners specific data analytical techniques. Such purposes are best served by entire courses in social statistics and biostatistics, with associated texts. Rather, a few useful suggestions will be offered regarding how to approach data within the context of a program evaluation.

Basic issues relevant to cost-benefit and cost-effectiveness analysis have already been presented in Chapter 3. The points raised below apply to such analysis as well as to any other experimental or quasi-experimental design that may have been employed. The basic concern is with overcoming the paralysis that frequently sets in when the evaluation team is suddenly confronted with data. "Analysis should never lead to paralysis" is a good dictum to follow. The following suggestions should assist the evaluator in making the dictum a reality.

First, it is important to consider data analysis issues early on in the design of the evaluation. How the data are to be analyzed depends on the program's objectives, the nature of the program itself, the particular evaluative design selected, the particular measures used, and the uses to which the data are likely to be put by various groups who will receive the evaluation report. For example, if there has been random assignment of subjects to experimental and control groups, there should be little need to include such variables as sex and age as "covariates" in an analysis of covariance model. Instead, a more straightforward analysis of variance may be employed. On the other hand, if a quasi-experimental design has been used (involving *nonrandomization* of subjects), it may be very important to take into account variables in which the two groups may differ (such as age, sex, race). This can be done by treating such variables as "covariates" within an analysis of covariance model.[16]

The concept of the effect of a covariate is illustrated in Table 10. Assume that we are evaluating the impact of an outreach program on increases in outpatient department utilization. Table 10 would tend to suggest that the outreach program had a significant effect on outpatient utilization, since 90 percent of those who received the program showed an increase in utilization of greater than 25 percent, while only 50 percent of those without the program showed such an increase. It could be that the difference can be accounted for not by the program but by differences in the composition of the two groups. One possibility is that the two groups differ by age. Age might therefore be considered a covariate and a possible alternative explanation for the results. In fact, Table 10 shows this to be the case. Those over 65 in *both* groups have higher utilization (eighty-five out of ninety in the experimental group, and eight out of ten in the comparison group). But, while ninety out of one hundred patients in the experimental group are over 65, only ten out of one hundred in the comparison group are over 65. Thus, there is strong evidence to suggest that the increased utilization may really be an effect of age rather than of the program itself. In brief, when age is taken into account as a covariate, the effects of the program disappear.

It is also important to emphasize that the type of data analysis will depend on the audience for whom the report is intended. For example, program officials, consumers, and public groups are likely to be most interested in the basic findings. In such cases a basic reporting of descriptive statistics (mean, standard deviation, and so on) may be sufficient. For other groups, such as outside evaluation consultants or fellow evaluators, greater interest may be

Table 10. Increase in outpatient utilization

	>25%	25% or less
Experimental group (received outreach program)	90%	10%
Comparison group (no outreach program)	50%	50%

	Over 65			Under 65		
	Total number	>25%	25% or less	Total number	>25%	25% or less
Experimental group	90	85	5	10	5	5
Comparison group	10	8	2	90	42	48

expressed in the more detailed and rigorous analysis. The important point to note is the need for *clear communication* in *language understandable* to the groups involved.

As a corollary to considering data analysis early in the design of the evaluation, one should feel free to seek expert statistical consultation. By bringing in such expertise early on, it is possible to avoid later pitfalls. Once the evaluator is attuned to thinking about data analysis as an integral and early part of the overall evaluation, several additional suggestions may be made. The first and most important is to "get close to the data." This means obtaining *first-hand knowledge of the distribution of each variable under study.* This is particularly important given the current widespread use of computers and the temptation to proceed to more sophisticated analysis without first obtaining a thorough understanding of the nature of the data. Close examination of basic distributions frequently provides leads for determining the choice of more advanced analytic methods. Analysis of distributions involves obtaining basic descriptive statistics such as the mean, standard deviation, range, kurtosis (a measure of skewness in the distribution), display of cumulative distributions, and, in some cases, plots of the data. Using such information, the evaluator can assess possible keypunch and coding errors, data outliers, and gaps in the data. For example, Fig. 9 shows a plot of the number of broken appointments of ten patients. Inspection of the data indicates that all patients except one have three or fewer broken appointments. The evaluator should be suspicious of individual No. 4, showing ten broken appointments. This is often called an "outlier." It may reflect an inaccurate reading of the office records from which the data were derived, a coding error, or a keypunch error. It should be checked out before it is accepted as valid. If its accuracy cannot be determined, it should be deleted from the analysis.

Plots can also be used to assess the extent to which the variables involved

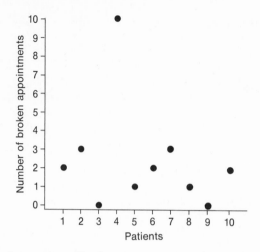

Fig. 9. Plot of patients and broken appointments (hypothetical example).

are normally distributed, and thus provide information regarding the possible need for various types of transformations. Problems of heteroscedasticity (where variable Y varies more for some values of variable X than for others) can be assessed.

Once the evaluator feels comfortable with the underlying nature of the data, *simple relationships* (using correlations or contingency tables) among the variables of interest should be examined. Again, it is tempting to proceed ahead to examination of multiple relationships, as in multiple regression, because most computer programs will print out the simple relationships among the variables (and, for that matter, descriptive statistics as well) at the same time that the simple relationships may reveal that several of the variables originally included in the multiple regression might have usefully been excluded, either because they are highly correlated with other independent variables in the model (the problem of multi-collinearity) or because virtually no relationship exists between a particular independent variable and the dependent variable of interest.

Inspection of sample contingency (cross-tabulation) tables may also reveal basic *interaction* effects that might be included in more sophisticated analyses. Using contingency tables, Table 11 provides an example of an interaction effect between race and patient satisfaction in regard to sex. Table 11 shows that whites are more likely to be satisfied than nonwhites (70 percent versus 30 percent). But it also shows that this relationship is particularly strong for females (90 percent of whites being highly satisfied versus only 10 percent of nonwhites), while no relationship exists at all for males (where an equal percentage of whites and nonwhites are highly satisfied). Failure to incorporate this interaction in the analysis might have led program administrators, providers, or planners to misinterpret the problem and propose irrelevant changes in organizational structure or program design. Since the results indicate that the problem arises only with nonwhite female patients, efforts at change should be tailored to that group.

Finally, regardless of the particular data analytical technique employed,

Table 11. Relationship between race and patient satisfaction

Race	Patient satisfaction	
	High	Low
White	70%	30%
Nonwhite	30%	70%

	Patient satisfaction (controlling for sex)			
	Female		Male	
Race	High	Low	High	Low
White	90%	10%	50%	50%
Nonwhite	10%	90%	50%	50%

emphasis needs to be given to the growing importance of *analyzing subgroups* and to *estimating the size of program effects.* Increasingly, program administrators and funding agencies are interested in knowing whether the program worked better with certain groups, perhaps based on age, sex, race, social class, geographic location, or health status, than for others, regardless of the overall impact of the evaluation. In such cases, given large enough sample sizes, the results should be broken out for each relevant subgroup, and separate analyses conducted within each subgroup. Furthermore, officials are interested not only in whether a program had an effect but in the degree of magnitude of the effect. For this purpose, greater use needs to be made of estimation techniques and computation of confidence intervals.[17]

Summary

This chapter has stressed the importance of measurement, data collection, and data analysis. Reliability was defined as the extent to which the same measure yields constant results on repeated applications; it is concerned with chance or random error. Validity was defined as the extent to which the measure reflects what it is supposed to measure. It is concerned with systematic error. A measure cannot be valid without also being reliable, but the reverse is not true; that is, it is possible for a measure to be reliable without being valid. Reliability and validity are particularly important to assess when dealing with new measures or new variables. A number of different methods for assessing reliability and validity were presented.

The importance of making use of existing archival or precollected data was stressed. These data can then be supplemented as needed by ongoing data collection efforts or questionnaires and interview data. The advantages and disadvantages of each were discussed. For most cases, a combination of all three methods is necessary.

Issues of data analysis need to be considered at an early point in the evaluation, and appropriate statistical consultation obtained. The importance of "getting close to one's data" was stressed by a thorough examination of basic descriptive statistics and simple relationships among variables. The importance of analyzing subgroup differences and estimating the magnitude of effects was also emphasized. Finally, one must keep in mind that most evaluations have multiple audiences interested in the report. Thus, it is necessary to use forms of analysis and report-writing that will be understandable to each group. Sometimes this can be done within the context of a single report but, frequently, it may require several different reports.

Chapters 3 and 4 have thus provided some basic technical material relevant to the design and execution of program evaluations. It is important to recognize that this material constitutes only a brief "waterfront" introduction to some difficult issues, particularly in regard to this chapter's material on measurement, data collection, and data analysis issues. Some of the more complex problems are covered in many of the readings suggested at the end of this chapter.

It is also important to recognize that such skills and knowledge are applied in dynamic operational settings and, because of this, frequently take on altered forms. Some of the pragmatic problems associated with conducting program evaluations as well as issues pertaining to program implementation itself are the subjects of Chapter 5.

Checklist of significant terms

Nominal measure	Convergent validity
Ordinal measure	Discriminant validity
Interval measure	Covariate
Ratio measure	Interaction effect
Reliability	Outlier
Validity	Contingency table

Sample problem exercises

1. In the study by Skipper and Leonard, briefly comment on the reliability and validity of each of the specific measures used in the study, namely, temperature, systolic blood pressure, pulse, emesis, voiding, fluid intake, nursing staff evaluation of control, and the mother's at-home evaluation. State whether or not you believe each of these is a reliable and valid measure, and why. For those measures about which you have some doubt, briefly suggest some additional reliability and validity checks you would like to see made.

2. Choose *any* concept involved in the Rand Health Insurance Experiment—mental health status, physical health status, patient satisfaction—and outline a multi-trait, multi-method approach to assessing the *reliability* and *validity* of a particular measure of the concept. Choose any measure of interest to you, but remember you are to design a multi-trait, multi-method approach to assessing the reliability and validity of that measure.

3. A measure can be reliable without being valid, but it is not possible to have a valid measure that is not also reliable.

State whether you agree or disagree with this statement and why. If you disagree, please give an example of a measure that is valid but not reliable.

4. You are responsible for conducting a study of patient satisfaction in the outpatient department of a large university hospital. You have your choice of using existing clinic data on broken appointments and expressed grievances, developing a self-administered questionnaire, conducting person-to-person interviews, or conducting telephone interviews. First, assume that a random sample of fifty patients is to be studied, and indicate your choice of data col-

lection and the reasons for your choice. Next, assume that a random sample of 500 patients is to be studied, and indicate your choice of data collection and reasons for your choice.

References

1. Cronbach, L.: Essentials of psychological testing, ed. 3, New York, 1970, Harper & Row, Publishers.
2. Campbell, D. T., and Fiske, D. W.: Convergent and discriminant validation by the multi-trait—multi-method matrix, Psychol. Bull. **56:**81-105, 1959.
3. Roos, N.: Evaluating health programs: where do we find the data? J. Community Health **1:**39-51, 1975.
4. Webb, E. J., and others: Unobtrusive measures: non-reactive research in the social sciences, Skokie, Ill., 1966, Rand McNally & Co.
5. Densen, P.: Epidemiologic contributions to health services research, Am. J. Epidemiol. 104:486-487, 1976.
6. Hodgson, D. A., and others: The uniform hospital discharge data demonstration: summary report, Washington, D.C., 1973, Department of Health, Education and Welfare, Health Resources Administration.
7. Robinson, J. P., and others: Measures of occupational attitudes and occupational characteristics, Ann Arbor, 1967, Survey Research Center, University of Michigan.
8. Robinson, J. P., and others: Measures of political attitudes, Ann Arbor, 1968, Survey Research Center, University of Michigan.
9. Robinson, J. P., and Shaver, P. R.: Measures of social/psychological attitudes, Ann Arbor, 1969, Survey Research Center, University of Michigan.
10. Shaw, M. E., and Wright, J. P.: Scales for the measurement of attitudes, New York, 1967, McGraw-Hill Book Co.
11. Price, J. P.: The handbook of organization measurement, Lexington, Mass., 1972, D. C. Heath & Co.
12. Aday, L., and Andersen, R.: The development of indices of access to medical care, Ann Arbor, 1975, Health Administration Press.
13. Sells, S. B., editor: The definition and measurement of mental health, Washington, D.C., 1968, Department of Health, Education and Welfare, National Center for Health Statistics.
14. Riedel, D., and others: Patient care evaluation in mental health programs, Cambridge, Mass., 1974, Ballinger Publishing Co.
15. Cobb, S., and Cannell, C. F.: Some thoughts about interview data, Int. Epidemiol. Assoc. Bull. **13:**43-54, 1966.
16. Campbell, D. T., and Stanley, J. C.: Experimental and quasi-experimental designs for research, Skokie, Ill., 1966, Rand McNally & Co. p. 23.
17. Hilton, E. H., and Lumsdaine, A. A.: Field trial designs in gauging the impact of fertility planning programs. In Bennett, C. A., and Lumsdaine, A. A., editors: Evaluation and experiment, New York, 1975, Academic Press, Inc., p. 396.

Suggested readings

Campbell, D. T., and Fiske, D. W.: Convergent and discriminant validation by the multi-trait—multi-method matrix, Psychol. Bull. **56:**81-105, 1959.
Dunn, O., and Clark, V.: Applied statistics: analysis of variance and regression, New York, 1974, John Wiley & Sons, Inc.
Moser, C. A., and Kalton, G.: Survey methods in social investigation, ed. 2, New York, 1972, Basic Books, Inc., Publishers, pp. 238-479.
National Center for Health Services Research: Advances in health survey research methods, Washington, D.C., 1975, Department of Health, Education and Welfare.
Riecken, H. W., and Boruch, R. F.: Social experimentation: a method for planning and evaluating social intervention, New York, 1974, Academic Press, Inc., pp. 117-152.
Roos, N.: Evaluating health programs: where do we find the data? J. Community Health **1:**39-51, 1975.
Suchman, E. A.: Evaluative research: principles and practice in public service and social action programs, New York, 1967, Russell Sage Foundation, pp. 115-131.
Walker, H. M., and Lev, J.: Statistical inference, New York, 1953, Holt, Rinehart and Winston, pp. 348-412.
Weiss, C.: Evaluation research: methods of assessing program effectiveness, Englewood Cliffs, N.J., 1972, Prentice-Hall, Inc., pp. 24-59.

CHAPTER 5 **Program evaluation and problems of implementation**

In previous chapters, a wide range of issues and methodologies for conducting program evaluations has been discussed. The emphasis has been on the task of the program evaluator. In this chapter, the relationship between health program evaluation and program implementation will be elaborated.

In the first section, a number of different settings within which evaluations typically take place will be described. These program settings range from the social experiment, such as the Rand Health Insurance Study, to ongoing health programs, such as evaluating the provision of school nursing services by a local health department, to the natural experiments, such as might be observed when a health insurance underwriter changes the nature of health benefits available to an enrolled population. Next, organizational issues will be discussed—for example, the range of actors or participants who may be involved in an overall program evaluation/program implementation effort. Third, the stages in the development of the program and its evaluation will be described. Fourth, issues of program implementation per se will be considered. And last, the relationship between the implementation of the evaluation and the implementation of the health program that is being evaluated will be closely examined.

Types of program settings

Whether health program evaluation constitutes the underlying rationale for conducting a major social experiment or, alternatively, is an ongoing function permanently established within a large health agency or institution, the activities and their results that are the subject of evaluation can typically be characterized as discrete programs ranging from the complex to the relatively simple. An evaluation team may work for several years attempting to determine the worth of a single large program and, equally important, the elements of the program that led to desired outcomes, anticipated but undesired outcomes, and unintended consequences. At the other extreme, a health program evaluation staff may undertake a series of evaluations of discrete programs sponsored by the agency, with each evaluation lasting only a few months, and sometimes with more than one evaluation being undertaken at one time. Program evaluation also differs in its intended audience, from federal to local, and in its source of funding. Since there is such a wide range of health programs that may be subject to evaluation, it is useful for our discussion of implementation issues and problems to classify program settings.

98

The social experiment

The social experiment may be viewed as a relatively self-contained type of field research intended to provide empirical evidence for a specific set of policy decisions. The principal, if not sole, purpose for undertaking the action program or intervention is to provide data for the program's evaluation. Thus, a heavy emphasis is placed on research design and its ability to provide answers to policy questions, with less emphasis placed on the preferences of providers or clients actually participating in the delivery or receipt of services.

In order to assure a satisfactory level of external validity, and indeed to assure satisfactory participation by professionals and clients in the action program, considerable attention needs to be paid to the design of the intervention itself. Nevertheless, the *raison d'être* of the action program as noted above is to provide data for the evaluation. Thus, in the myriad of decisions that need to be made in the course of designing and executing the social experiment, conflicts will, to the degree possible, be resolved in favor of the integrity of the research effort.

Demonstration projects

Demonstration projects typically differ from social experiments in that they are not viewed as being inherently bounded by their value to research on social questions or by a clear-cut end-point once the results of the intervention are known. Rather, the demonstration project from the outset is more likely to take on the character of a prototype, and formative evaluation is often the approach that is employed. The evaluation component of the demonstration project, while not as central to its purpose as in the case of the social experiment, is viewed as an essential ingredient. Some federal agencies will not provide funding unless the project has a strong evaluation plan, on the grounds that in the absence of such a plan what is proposed would be strictly a service project and therefore not eligible for funding.

While social experiments are commonly conceived by a central agency which maintains close working relationships with the evaluation team, demonstration projects are more often the result of local initiative. Many sites may be funded to increase the geographic distribution of the program, thus improving its chances of widespread adoption. Application is usually made within the framework of state or federal guidelines, and multiple projects are funded on a competitive basis. The amount of attention given to program evaluation may be considerably less than one would observe in the first case, particularly if the agency guidelines indicate that evaluation is an adjunct to program operations rather than the funding agency's principal intent.

A good example of the latter case is the Office of Economic Opportunity (OEO) neighborhood health center program which was developed as one of the Great Society undertakings of the 1960s. The neighborhood health center movement grew out of the broader community action program thrust of OEO. The delivery of health services emerged as a particularly attractive vehicle through which to develop community action at the local level. It had face validity as a social program, could provide services that were applicable to the entire community, and provided a structured if not well-understood meeting ground for clients and professionals. As the appeal of neighborhood health centers became more widely recognized, appropriations for the Office of Health Affairs, OEO, increased. The major emphasis of applications coming from various sponsors around the country, however, clearly emphasized the service component as an innovative way of solving many of the health care problems facing poor populations. By and large, the evaluation activity was imposed on these center grantees, with funding coming out of their operating budgets. Under these circumstances, it can be seen that evaluation personnel would play a role secondary to the action component.

Developmental programs

Even more appropriate for the use of formative evaluation techniques is the developmental program. In contrast to the larger scale demonstration project, developmental programs characteristically are locally developed, individual prototypes intended to test an innovative idea. The testing phase determines whether the idea will work in practice or, after considerable trial and error, under what circumstances the idea can be put into practice.

Because of the exploratory nature of developmental programs and their great diversity, there is no established pattern in the relationships between evaluation and program implementation. There is considerable merit, however, in early consultation between the innovator and an experienced evaluator. This is true for at least three reasons. First, the developmental program leader will typically be more interested in the implementation process per se than in documenting it. Second, it is unlikely that the innovator will have the necessary training or experience to undertake a useful and objective formative appraisal; and third, valuable data will be lost if the evaluator, even if serving only in a consulting capacity, is not involved early in the process.

New program implementation

Many ongoing institutions and agencies, particularly in the public sector, formalize the addition of major new *services* by describing them as new *programs* to be added to the existing range of services. In the hospital setting, it might be a self-care unit or a patient education program. In a community health agency, a new program might consist of alcoholism counseling services or emergency medical services. These programs may be based on an earlier developmental project in some other setting. Before the agency commits itself to integrating the new program into its accepted range of ongoing services to the community, there will often be external or internal pressures for an evaluation of the program's worth.

A common problem in the evaluation of new programs is that the program is not fully thought through at the outset and may be modified as unforeseen, but inevitable, factors impinge upon implementation. Because of this, the original evaluation plan may prove to be impractical, or the evaluative data that are generated may not be relevant to assessing the program as it was actually carried out.

Modification of an ongoing program

In contrast to the four cases cited, program evaluation may be undertaken in the situation where changes are to be made in an existing program. New methods of organization, new therapeutic techniques, a new clientele, or, in the extreme, even justification of current activities may represent the substance of the evaluation activity. It is in the evaluation of this type of intervention that the evaluator has the least direct control over the action component and must be most skillful in recognizing potential pitfalls. In a large agency or institution, the modification of an existing program or introduction of "innovative methods" may be stimulated by external review or simply by management's dissatisfaction with the existing system.

The modified approach is (1) most often conceived or at least originally endorsed by a higher level in the organization, (2) in response to a desire to "find a better way, " and (3) intended to produce measurable results that may affect other components of the organization in the future. Thus considerable emphasis is likely to be placed on evaluation. At the same time, such an evaluation provides a potential threat to professional personnel in the organization who are accustomed to established patterns of behavior. The use of outside consultants is common both for the design of such an evaluation and for assistance in modifying the existing program.

The natural experiment

Retrospective evaluation of major changes in health programs is becoming increasingly popular. Less common, but still important, is the concurrent or even prospective assessment of such changes. The natural experiment, then, is the situation in which the change is made without regard to its evaluation but occurs in such a way as to allow the investigator to make inferences and draw conclusions on the basis of comparative data. This type of intervention is "natural" in the sense that the intervention is independent of evaluation, but it is called an "experiment" because it was carried out in such a way as to allow for a valid comparison to assess the impact of the change.

Under these circumstances, the program evaluator has usually not participated in the implementation of the intervention and must make judgments about internal and external validity not for the purpose of design, but rather for the purpose of deciding whether the natural experiment is worth analyzing. The most common problem encountered with this type of program evaluation, once the natural design is considered sufficiently valid to warrant analysis, is inadequate data. The program evaluator must take special pains to be sure the changes that were made, and the degree to which they can be isolated from external events, are clearly understood.

Organizational issues

Several major organizational issues must be considered in the light of the wide range of program settings. The first is the variation in the composition of the "evaluation team" and the "action team" as one compares types of programs to be evaluated. Second is the variation that occurs in the relationship between these teams. The third area, which can also be viewed according to setting, concerns administrative relationships. And the fourth major issue has to do with the question of operations. Discussion of this fourth consideration will be deferred to the last section of the chapter, which deals with the synchronization of a health program and its evaluation.

Range of participants

In the preceding section, reference was made to the "evaluation team" and the "action team." The size and complexity of these two groups depend on the type of intervention or program; the complexity of either the intervention or the evaluation, or both; and the nature of the organization within which the program and its evaluation are taking place. For example, a social experiment such as the Rand Health Insurance Study has a substantial number of key senior individuals on both "teams," with action or program personnel located in multiple sites. At the other extreme, in the retrospective natural experiment, there would typically be only the evaluation team, or perhaps only a single evaluator. Finally, an important characteristic of program evaluation, as opposed to most health services research, is the importance and ongoing role of the sponsor.

In some instances, the sponsor will also be the primary user of the evaluation results. In other cases, however, the sponsor may be a higher level in the organization or a federal funding agency, while the intended audience is a legislative body. In addition, program personnel may be explicitly included in the audience or user group. For example, the evaluation of a change in method of delivering services within an ongoing program might be sponsored by a higher level in the agency or institution to determine whether the new technique should be applied more broadly. At the same time, program personnel can learn (from data provided by the evaluation project) under what circumstances the new technique proved to be most effective, or what program elements did not seem to improve the process of care or the well-being of patients.

The evaluation team typically comprises a "principal investigator" and at least one additional individual to assist with field operations. In a relatively simple evaluation, the principal investigator or program evaluator may be responsible for designing the evaluation, including developing measurement instruments such as questionnaires or other data collection forms, supervising data collection, analyzing the data, and reporting. Actual data collection would most often be the responsibility of a staff member. For more complex evaluations, a number of professionals may have specialized tasks for design, development of methods, data preparation and processing, and analysis and reporting. Data collection may involve a large-scale field operation with one or more field supervisors. It is not unusual to draw on consultants for the more technical aspects of design, measurement and data collection, and analysis.

The action team typically encompasses the functions of program development (or design of the intervention itself), program management, and professional performance. These functions may be carried out by three different individuals or groups of individuals. For example, a behavior modification program for families of children with learning disorders to be introduced by a hospital outpatient department might include a psychiatrist responsible for the design of the program, another member of the department responsible for the day-to-day management of the program and staff, and professional staff responsible for carrying out the intervention. As in the case of the program evaluation, there may be considerable dependence on outside consultants for program design and development.

Interrelationships between teams

We have seen that there is a range of settings within which programs may be evaluated and considerable variation in the complexity of both the evaluation team and the action team. An important dimension along which to array different types of programs is the degree of control that the program evaluator has over the implementation and operation of the program itself.

The extreme case is the *social experiment,* with its emphasis on providing evaluative results. Unlike other types of programs typically subject to evaluation, the senior management of the social experiment, as well as both evaluation and project leadership, are generally the full responsibility of the evaluator. In the *demonstration project,* the applicant will most often be the head of the action team. Thus, in contrast to the social experiment, the individual responsible for the demonstration's evaluation is usually found in a secondary role.

The evaluator typically exerts even less influence in the evaluation of *developmental programs* or *new program implementations.* While evaluation is important in both cases, particularly for the purpose of future acceptance of the innovation or new program, there seems to be a much clearer distinction between the role of the evaluation team and the role of the action team. One usually observes greater organizational distance between the individuals responsible for the action program and those responsible for the evaluation program. In a sense, the evaluator has less control over the design and the execution of the program itself than he would have in the earlier two instances discussed, and there is greater opportunity for suspicion and distrust between the two teams. The implications of weaker ties between evaluators and program personnel will be discussed more fully later.

When the evaluation is undertaken to assess *modifications of ongoing programs,* there is both greater organizational distance between the evaluation team and the action team, as was true in the previous case, and also greater incentive for the action team to formulate platitudinous objectives while actually departing as little as possible from their accustomed way of doing things. Andrew, reporting on four cases of experimental programs designed to introduce a new approach in an ongoing public agency, cites a number of "stresses" that can develop in this situation. These will be described in more detail later. Suffice it to say here that few stresses were noted as a result of personal characteristics and interpersonal relationships. Rather, the major stresses could be summarized as, "(1) those which were inherent in the *managerial arrangements* of the project, and (2) those growing out of program and research demands and their interaction, labeled the *professional context.*"[1]

Finally, we consider the *natural experiment*. With this type of evaluation the program evaluator almost by definition has little or no control over the intervention. The major relationships that must be developed with project personnel are for purposes of thoroughly understanding exactly what the intervention was and obtaining sufficient data to be able to assess the program's impact.

Administrative relationships

In a social experiment the functions of evaluation design, on the one hand, and program design and development, on the other, are closely intertwined. Similarly, there is usually a stronger collaborative relationship in implementation than is found in other types of programs. Demonstration projects and programs in large agencies or institutions present a more ambiguous picture in terms of responsibility for evaluation and working relationships between the evaluation team and the action team. The principle that personnel responsible for conducting a program should not be responsible for its formal evaluation is widely accepted. The credibility of an evaluation in which this principle is not followed would be questioned for a number of reasons that are themselves related to the difficulties encountered in the relationships between program evaluation and program implementation. We will turn next to these relationships.

Even if one assumes the most favorable interpersonal relationships, the program evaluation team is bound to be at odds with the action team to some degree from start to finish. A number of factors can be identified that are present in almost all situations. Mechanic clearly states one of the most fundamental factors:

> In considering varying social policies, the more rigorous evaluation research-
> er tends to focus on behavioral outcomes and, thus, assumes a relatively
> conservative stance. For example, it is typical for such persons to maintain
> that if a particular social intervention has not been proven effective, then pub-
> lic programs should not extend such services. In contrast, both administrators
> of intervention programs and the interested public may value a service—not
> because it has with some degree of frequency objectively altered behavior in a
> desired direction—but because it has been deemed valuable in the society
> more generally and provides a sense of security or reduces a subjective sense
> of discomfort.[2]

Beyond this rather basic philosophical difference, there are a number of very practical psychological and administrative differences in perspective that can be identified. First, evaluation is expensive and, at least at the outset, the usefulness of the results are often questioned by the action team. When funds are explicitly diverted from the delivery of services to provide support for the evaluation, as in the OEO neighborhood health center instance described earlier, the action team is likely at least to question the allocation of resources if not to resent this diversion of funds. This problem arises, however, even when evaluation funds are allocated from a separate and distinct source rather than diverted from service delivery. Second, design of the program evaluation, including measurement, directly impinges on the conduct of the program itself. The evaluation may require the action team to spend time completing forms, to follow a protocol that seems unnatural to them, or to defer making changes during the course of the evaluation that would appear to improve patient care or be more efficient. Third, the evaluation team may be viewed as having special privileges and not subject to the usual constraints of the organization. For example, close contact may be maintained between the program evaluator and higher levels of the organization or the funding agency. Furthermore, the evaluator may be seen as free to intervene and then move on to another project without having to bear responsibility for the less attractive drudgery of day-to-day service delivery. Fourth, the role of the evaluator calls for objectivity and a degree of skepticism. In contrast, the very success of the action team may depend on unrestrained commitment and enthusiasm. Riecken and Boruch have noted:

> It is a very rude awakening for the qualitatively-minded laissez-faire oriented action agent to submit his practices to the review and test of research procedures that seem unsympathetic or hostile. Research procedures often challenge the action agent's conviction (on the basis of his intuition and experience) that his skills will produce intended effects. It seems strange to the practitioner that the efficacy of his techniques are, perhaps for the first time, not accepted as self-evident. The researcher's scientific objectivity becomes viewed as inappropriate, somehow unfair, and threatening.[3]

These observers go on to point out that more than the action team egos may be involved. An unfavorable evaluation may result in an adverse impact on careers, as well as on continuation of the program or project.

A fifth and related factor is value differences. The program evaluator is committed to maintaining the integrity of the design. His value commitment is to scientific study. By contrast, the action team is service-oriented.

> Ideologically, action practitioners are committed to respond when they encounter someone who needs their services. To tell them that they are to serve only every fourth or tenth person in need; or that they are to treat only those on one side of the street and not the other; to tell them *not* to help the controls even if sufficient treatment resources are available for allocation to nonexperimental eligibles—seems inhumane and contrary to their basic purpose in life.[3]

While these conflicts between the evaluation team and the action team are present in most situations, there are steps that can be taken to minimize the amount of conflict. Considerable weight should be given to allowing time for discussion of differences and the development of mutual understanding. In addition, however, clear communication of different types of goals, management support for both evaluation and program personnel apart from the evaluation process, and attention to the needs of patients assigned to comparison or control groups outside the framework of the evaluation design will improve the climate within which health program evaluation takes place. Some of these factors will be considered in the section on the coordination of evaluation and program implementation.

Stages in program development and evaluation

Whatever the type of program to be evaluated, it can be viewed as a change in the way of doing things that arises from a perception that the present approach to diagnosis, treatment, organization of services, or financing is not socially optimal and can be improved. As D'Costa and Sechrest point out, "Experimentation with new systems is . . . an important responsibility of the health administrator. Any time there is concern with an existing system and new ones are to be tried out, evaluation is the instrument of choice to justify the ultimate implementation of such change."[4] These authors go on to lay out a useful model for program evaluation. Their approach forms the basis for assessing the usefulness of an intervention in meeting societal needs. The D'Costa and Sechrest model suggests that certain kinds of questions need to be addressed:

1. What is the setting in which the program is to be implemented?
2. What are the problems for redress or what improvements should the program aim at?
3. What are some good strategies to achieve these aims? What resources are available?
4. How well have we utilized the resources available?
5. What outcomes have we achieved? Not achieved? What unintended outcomes or side effects have been obtained?
6. Are these outcomes worthwhile? What impact have we had on society?
7. How could the program have been implemented better?
8. What policy changes would society benefit from?[4]

These broad questions underlie a "natural progression of steps" that are found in essentially any complete evaluation program. They may also be thought of in terms of stages which have been diagrammed by D'Costa and Sechrest as shown in Fig. 10. This figure provides a further elaboration of the basic evaluation process shown earlier in Fig. 2 (p. 17). The outer circle represents corresponding program objectives and design, analysis of program functioning, outcomes as measured by the specific evaluation design, and recommendations arising from the program evaluation.

The D'Costa and Sechrest model is a useful framework for considering both program implementation and the implementation of a program evaluation. The societal components or stages (numbers 1, 4, 6, and 8) are particularly concerned with the original impetus for programmatic change, external validity, and the ultimate usefulness of the program (whether it be a social experiment or a specific change within an ongoing program). The first stage, social needs or contexts, is concerned with the conditions leading to programmatic intervention and such characteristics of the setting as professional arrangements, client characteristics, and related factors.

The importance of this stage may be illustrated by considering evaluation of a utilization review program in two hospitals. In the first case, one might imagine a tight bed supply in a particular community and resultant waiting periods for elective surgical admissions. In the second hospital, one might find much lower occupancy rates and no delay in admitting patients for any condition. Under the former circumstance, it would be in the interests of all concerned (hospital administration, medical staff members, and the community) to institute a tight utilization review program that would assure early discharge of patients whenever possible to free a bed for use by the patient of another physician. The success of the utilization review program might be well documented in the first hospital. In the case of the second hospital, however, what would appear to be the same program might have no impact on reduced length of stay. If the programs were mandated by an external organization, such as the state Medicaid program, the rationale from a societal point of view could be seen as reducing the fiscal burden of the state. This, however, is

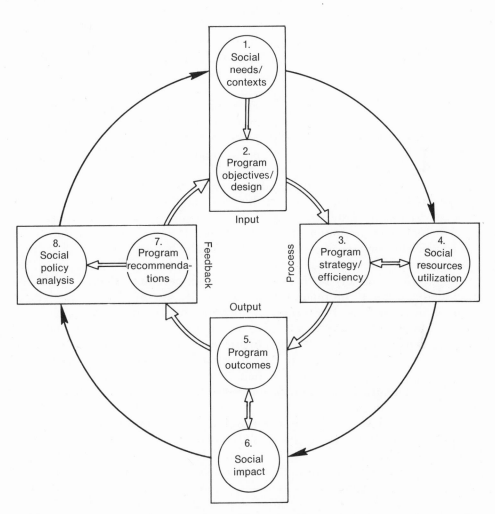

Fig. 10. Stages in program evaluation. (From D'Costa, A., and Sechrest, L.: Program evaluation concepts for health administrators, Washington, D.C., Association of University Programs in Health Administration, 1976.)

not sufficient motivation for the parties directly involved to ensure program success. Careful consideration of the context within which the program is being implemented would reveal that, as designed, it would be effective only if the interests of the outside agency coincided with the interests of the personnel responsible for program implementation. Thus, the success of the program in the first hospital could not be generalized.

Although not discussed in detail by D'Costa and Sechrest, the fourth stage of social resources utilization is useful to consider in program implementation and program evaluation implementation because of the constraints that might be placed on program strategy and/or efficiency. For example, in a neighborhood health center program, improved efficiency might in part depend on a small and experienced governing board. However, program maintenance within a particular political climate might dictate broader representation from various groups within a community. Such a strategy may not contribute to the organization's primary goals but may, on the other hand, be important to the attainment of social goals that transcend the particular program or organization.

The sixth stage described by D'Costa and Sechrest, and the third element in the evaluation process relating the program to the social system, is called social impact appraisal. It is at this point that the results of the program are viewed in the context of the originally perceived organizational or social needs. The program may have been carried out in a way that closely followed the original design and produced the outcomes that were hoped for as a result of a new intervention. If this is the case, and the social and political context has not changed substantially, then the results of the social experiment, demonstration, or programmatic intervention will provide the basis on which policy decision-makers may proceed. More likely, however, any or all of these elements will have changed over time. New opportunities arising in the health services delivery setting or unanticipated program outcomes will have provided additional information that may modify the original conceptualization of the program. For example, difficulty in recruiting physicians in sufficient number to provide effective monitoring for a utilization review system may lead to the substitution of nursing personnel using criteria developed by physicians. This approach, in turn, may have led to sharper specification of criteria by physicians, more immediate feedback to medical staff members, and, ultimately, the idea of concurrent rather than retrospective review to improve effectiveness of physician response.

Finally, the last step in the health program evaluation process is the dissemination of information gathered throughout the program implementation and program evaluation stages in a form that is useful for decision-makers within the program and within the sponsoring organization, and for other audiences engaged in policy decision-making. As will be noted below, this can be a demanding and time-consuming stage that is often neglected as program administrators and evaluators shift attention to some new undertaking.

The preceding paragraphs summarize the stages of program implementation and evaluation with respect to their social context. For each of these there is a corresponding element or stage more directly related to program implementation per se. These are shown in the inner circle of Fig. 10. At the second stage, the general program strategy is translated into specific goals and objectives. The action team may be reluctant to specify particular target groups, methods of intervention, or desired outcomes. However, as previously noted (Chapter 2), it is important for the program evaluator to be able to specify observable and measurable behaviors. More will be said of this later.

The third stage entails developing and implementing the program design—that is, choosing among the wide range of possible interventions, whether they be coinsurance rates, configurations of health teams, choice of educational methods or contents, or particular diagnostic or therapeutic techniques. It is at this stage, for example, that the evaluator carefully describes the manner in which the program operates and the changes that occurred over the course of the intervention.

The fifth stage in the overall evaluation process, and the third programmatic step, is the analysis of outcomes, both intended and unintended. Several of the previous chapters have directly addressed this stage.

Finally, the results of the program, both in its implementation and its outcome, need to be analyzed and reported. It is this report that will be used by other professionals considering adoption of the intervention that has been undertaken. This stage precedes and is not the same as the broader diffusion of information arising from the program and its evaluation.

In the following section, some of the difficulties of program implementation per se will be considered. Then, within the framework of these stages of evaluation, the issues and problems that arise in the coordination of program implementation and evaluation implementation will be examined.

Program implementation

Even experienced administrators tend to underestimate the complexity and time requirements of a new program. This may be due in part to external pressures, which in turn arise from the widespread lack of understanding on the part of policy-makers and constituencies of the demands of program implementation. Surprisingly little systematic attention has been paid to the questions of why the actual results of new programs or major changes in ongoing programs often bear little resemblance to the original intent of policy-makers, are frequently delayed, and usually are far more modest than initially envisioned.

It is popular to assert that the originators in their enthusiasm overpromised (perhaps intentionally) what could be accomplished. It is also widely believed that influential opponents intervene to radically alter or actually thwart implementation of new programs or program changes. Finally, bureaucracy is viewed as a villain in the effective implementation of new programs or program changes. While there may be more than a grain of truth present in all these explanations for a given program, they are not necessary. Rather, it is striking how often ordinary, well-accepted perceptions, working relationships, inter-agency arrangements, and day-to-day procedures accumulate to make implementation exceedingly difficult.

Considering first the perceptions of various actors, Williams identifies two partially overlapping spheres of action: policy and operations.[5] Persons in the policy sphere are concerned with major governmental (or organizational) directions and resource allocation decisions. Their attention tends to move from program to program, with personal and organizational rewards measured in terms of the success of getting a program launched or the amount of resources controlled. Williams notes:

> When a program moves toward the field, these policymakers tend to lose interest. More accurately, they are interested if events occur which push program issues back into the policy sphere. If something happens in the field that raises the ire of an important congressman, agency policymakers are immediately concerned. However, their concern is not with the often tedious activities that carry the program from level to level, and finally to an operating entity, which may have the greatest power to affect participants in the program. Yet it is in this mundane world that power in the sense of effect may be found. At some point far down in the process, away from the policy sphere, people can bungle things badly, and their mistakes probably will go relatively unnoticed by those concerned with "big" policy issues. Of course, the consequence is that things do not work out as policymakers planned. This is why power and powerlessness can exist together.[5]

The rewards, then, for persons in the policy sphere are not closely related to how efficiently the program was implemented or even how closely the outcome reflects the original intent. At the same time, there is a strong tendency for those charged with implementation at various levels of an organization to place more emphasis on their relationships with persons closer to the policy sphere than with those more concerned with operations. The rewards of implementation are limited in most large organizations, particularly governmental. Furthermore, the tasks are typically diffused with inadequate attention to management responsibility. The result is that as program implementation moves from higher levels in the organization where general guidelines are developed to regional offices (as in the federal government) or operating sites where day-to-day decisions are made, it is easy for the perceptions of the "action team" to deviate widely from the original intent of the policy decisionmakers who initiated the program or program change.

In addition to the common problems that arise from lack of emphasis on systematic implementation within large social agencies or health organizations, implementation is further complicated by the frequent involvement of multiple organizations and individual medical care providers. For example, most federal health programs depend on voluntary organizations to actually provide the services and may channel the funds through subnational governments, or contract with state agencies to perform the function of certification of eligible providers.

The dependence on multiple state and local organizations creates at least two types of fundamental problems for program implementation, which may appear in modified form even within a single complex delivery organization, such as a hospital. First, as Mechanic has noted, "even when the intent of a program is clearly specified at the highest administrative levels, the translations at the local units can be quite bizarre; and the operational units tend to have their own agendas and priorities and often quite diverse goals."[2] Local units or professionals may be participating for a variety of reasons quite unrelated to the overall intent of the program. Second, coordination among participating agencies or providers is expensive and time-consuming, and often insufficient resources are devoted to its accomplishment. Because participants often have other responsibilities and activities, program implementation typically does not move forward without specific and more or less continuous attention on the part of a lead agency or individual.

Two brief examples may help to illustrate these problems of multiple agendas and coordination. Elinson and Herr contrast the stated national intent in establishing OEO neighborhood health centers with some of the latent functions of these centers as viewed from the local level.[6] The former was to provide comprehensive ambulatory health services of high quality, which could be coordinated with other community services, and to emphasize consumer involvement. A partial list of latent functions, stated or perceived at the local level, implied quite different objectives:

1. Improving the image of the black male in poverty communities
2. Stimulating and maintaining solidarity among migrant Chicano farm workers
3. Pacification of hostile communities by colonial powers
4. Discharging missionary service obligations of the medical-hospital establishment
5. Filling a political void in social and economic action
6. Politicization or radicalization of youth

The contrast does not necessarily indicate incompatible objectives, but simply illustrates one kind of difficulty that arises in program implementation.

The second example is found in the masterful analysis by Pressman and Wildavsky of a major set of Economic Development Agency public works programs implemented in Oakland, California. These programs involved no conspicuous conflicting interests, contradictory legislative criteria, lack of funding, or local opposition. The failure of the program is fascinating and instructive just because it appears so straightforward. As the authors observe, "What is so hard about building a terminal and airline hangar when the money is there, the plans are signed, and the people agree that minorities are to get a share of the jobs?"[7] The analysis goes on to illustrate that in fact the numerous participants, perspectives, clearances, and other decision points accumulate in such a way as to make implementation exceedingly complex, due to the many opportunities for disagreement and delay. Delay is viewed as a function of the intensity of interest in any particular decision that is needed, as well as whether the decision-maker is favorably or unfavorably inclined. Delay in one area, of course, affects other facets of implementation. Apart from delay, however, one needs only to consider that if a program needs just seven agreements or clearances and the independent probability of obtaining each one is .9, the odds of successful implementation are less than 50-50.

Finally, it should be noted that with delay and lack of coordination, earlier agreements or understandings tend to erode, key actors leave, and new circumstances begin to influence decision-makers. Thus, the issues of program implementation, while seeming mundane in some respects, are a critical factor to be taken into account in health program evaluation.

Relation of program to evaluation implementation

In this final section, a number of problems that have been touched on throughout the chapter will be discussed further within the context of synchronized implementation of a health program and its evaluation. It is clear that there is a wide range of programs or program changes that may be subject to evaluation, and, further, that the relationships between the evaluation team and the action team differ systematically as a function of the nature of the program. It has also been noted that there are some natural sources of friction between these two teams in most situations. Because of the complexity of these factors, coupled with inevitable problems of implementation per se, it is difficult to talk in general terms about the specific problems of linking program implementation and evaluation implementation. Nevertheless, there are problems and suggested solutions that are sufficiently generic to warrant specific consideration and appreciation. These may be most usefully examined within the framework of the evaluation model described above and shown in Fig. 10.

Let us first consider the transition from the first to the second stage of the D'Costa and Sechrest model, in which the general program strategy is translated into specific goals and objectives. As noted earlier, the action team may not wish to specify target groups, methods of intervention, or desired outcomes in sufficient detail to satisfy the needs of the program evaluator for observable and measurable behaviors that can be included in an evaluation design.

The difficulty of obtaining clearly specified program goals arises from a number of factors that were alluded to earlier. First, the sheer complexity and pressure arising from program implementation often leaves little time for careful thought regarding the needs of the evaluation team. Furthermore, as in the case of legislation, which is often the product of compromise among competing interests, the action team may not wish to exacerbate difficulties in achieving consensus among various participants by sharply defining goals and objectives. Rather, generalities may serve a useful political purpose.

Evaluators should be concerned both with obtaining specification of goals that are sufficiently clear to be subject to evaluation and also with the forces at work that make agreement on goals difficult. That is, the evaluator should be concerned with not only outcome measures but also those factors that influence the program's likelihood to achieve the outcome.

As previously noted (Chapter 2), Weiss suggests that the best approach is to set up a collaborative effort with the action team in the formulation of goals. "Sitting with the program people, the evaluator can offer successive approximations of goal statements. The program staff modifies them, and the discussion continues until agreement is reached."[8] This approach has the advantage of recognizing that new programs, as well as program changes, are often evolutionary because of the difficulties of implementation. It is particularly important in evaluating program changes to recognize the value of considering a dynamic program evaluation strategy. For example, the evaluator should be prepared to have a sufficient number of measures on various elements of the program to anticipate possible shifts in goals as the program and its environment adapt to changes over time and to be able to identify and describe changes in the means by which goals are achieved.

In addition, the evaluator must be able to distinguish between situations in which clearer specification of goals will be a productive exercise in both achieving true consensus among action team participants and providing a basis for the evaluation, and in which premature closure on goals may not only be disruptive to the program but may actually distort the original intent by causing the action team to pursue measures of success that inadequately reflect the major program elements. An example of the former might be the case in which a hospital self-care unit is intended to reduce the number of nursing personnel employed by a hospital, as well as to provide a more suitable environment for appropriate patients. An example of the latter might be the goal of reducing duplication of capital expenditures in hospitals within a community as measured by the volume of proposed expenditures that are denied by the local health planning agency. It can be seen that in this case the measure may become the goal. Of much greater interest to policy decision-makers would probably be the effects of the health planning agencies' criteria and review procedures on the behavior of hospitals that were contemplating new capital expenditures.

In the more tightly structured situation in which the evaluation is a major component—for example, the social experiment or demonstration project—one still finds difficulty in defining the goals with sufficient precision to satisfy the requirements of the program evaluator. Apart from the problems associated with implementation referred to above, one often finds fear of failure contributing to reluctance on the part of the action team. Two points are particularly pertinent in this regard. First, an experienced evaluator will emphasize the underlying conceptual model which is being tried out in practice. If the action team is encouraged to think more broadly about what it is doing, standards of judging relative success or failure can probably be agreed upon ahead of time. This matter becomes very important when the results are in and being interpreted for the sponsor or the policy decision-makers. Second, focusing on the model helps to clarify the distinctions among ultimate, intermediate, and immediate objectives, previously discussed in Chapter 2.

It will be recalled that *ultimate objectives* refer to the end-result that the program is intended to produce, for example, lower age-adjusted blood pressure. *Intermediate objectives* refer to the programmatic means to be employed to achieve the ultimate objectives, such as improving continuity of care. And *immediate objectives* refer to the specific operational procedures that must be carried out to implement the program (for example, hire a nurse practitioner).

It is, of course, essential to measure immediate objectives to adequately describe the "treatment." More important for the purpose of this discussion, however, is the fact that some of the anxiety surrounding evaluation can be dissipated if the evaluator makes clear to the action team that the program can fail even though the specified procedures (immediate objectives) are carried out in an exemplary fashion. In other words, as noted in Chapter 2, if the action team understands that a failure of theory is going to be distinguished from failure to carry out their jobs, and, further, that the programmatic intervention is being tested and not their technical or professional competence, then some fears might be alleviated. This suggestion is by no means a complete resolution of the difficulty, because the action team almost by definition will find it very difficult not to be fully committed to the success of "their program."

The next phase is the transition from specifying goals to developing and implementing a particular program design. In the earlier section on organizational issues, several areas of conflict between the action team and the evaluation team were described. It was noted that strong management support for both evaluation and program personnel was required to improve the climate within which health program evaluation takes place. Further, common issues such as accommodating to changes in the environment and, more generally, dealing with the inevitable tendency for the program to shift course, are all important problems of implementation.

For some types of program evaluation, such as the social experiment at one extreme or the natural experiment at the other, management responsibility is more or less clear-cut. In the majority of cases falling in the middle ground, however, there is considerable opportunity for confusion. In the large health organization or agency, for example, the chief executive officer has ultimate responsibility for program evaluation that takes place within his jurisdiction. Attention must be given to providing sufficient staffing of both the action team and the evaluation team to ensure that their efforts can move ahead in synchronization and that the pressures of program implementation do not lead to inappropriate use of evaluation personnel for day-to-day program operations. Management involvement in overseeing program evaluation activities clearly increases the likelihood of the results having an impact on organizational change.

The requirement that the evaluation team be independent of the program being evaluated has been mentioned in terms of the future credibility and usefulness of results. There is another very practical factor to be considered, however, in terms of implementation. Health program evaluation projects are time-limited and, in most instances, require specialized staff who, except in the largest agencies, will not be permanent employees. Particularly in institutions and agencies with complex personnel systems (such as the Civil Service), it is very important that substantial lead-time be allowed and that management obtain as much flexibility in recruitment as possible. As Andrew notes, "The trick is to convey the idea that the project is special and, therefore, recruitment and salaries are exempt from those prevailing *but* the special nature is *not* a question of higher status. Rather, it is based on the time-limited aspects and consequent recruitment problems."[1] Andrew goes on to observe that

Unfortunately it is almost a point of honor for a project director not to attend to problems of this order because they are administrative and not scientific questions. Nevertheless, he will be fortunate if he can recruit a project staff within six months after his grant has begun even when he makes the suggested preparations. Failure to do so can extend that period to much of the effective time of the grant and further, if these problems are not resolved, they will constantly intrude on his time throughout the project period.[1]

The problem of delayed implementation is as much a problem for the action team as it is for the evaluation team. One common problem often overlooked in preliminary planning for health program evaluation is the startup period during which sample sizes are insufficient to meet the evaluation design requirements and, in addition, procedures have not been fully tried out to ensure proper randomization or other design requirements. It is often useful to explicitly establish a trial period during which both program and evaluation procedures can be worked out before moving into the formal study period.

Once the program and its evaluation are in the field, many pressures for change will arise both externally and internally. This happens for many reasons, including shifts in social objectives of the sponsoring agency (such as greater integration into other community-delivery systems or cost containment), unanticipated changes in levels of funding, and turnover among senior personnel, to name a few. Weiss offers several suggestions on how the program evaluator can best cope with program drift:

1. Take frequent periodic measures of program effect (for example, monthly assessments in program of education, training, therapy) rather than limiting collection of outcome data to one point in time.
2. Encourage a clear transition from one program approach to another. If changes are going to be made, try to see that A is done for a set period, then B, then C.
3. Clarify the assumptions and procedures of each phase and classify them systematically.
4. Keep careful records of the persons who participated in each phase. Rather than lumping all participants together, analyze outcomes in terms of the phase(s) of program in which each person participated.
5. Press for a recycling of earlier program phases. Sometimes this happens naturally; on occasion, it can be engineered. If it is possible, it provides a way to check on earlier conclusions.
6. Seek to set aside funds and get approval for smaller-scale evaluation of a given period. For this venture, experimental procedures can be applied, even though less rigorous and more flexible methods may be sufficient in other program areas.
7. If nothing works and the program continues to meander (chaos would be the proper word in some contexts), consider jettisoning the evaluation framework in favor of meticulous analysis of the what, how, and why of events.[8]

One element in the evaluation process that is not formally incorporated into the D'Costa and Sechrest model is the ongoing assessment of the evaluation effort itself. It is often useful, for example, to establish regularly scheduled reviews of the evaluation by outside consultants. A second factor that also needs regular monitoring is the degree to which the evaluation process or preliminary results might be influencing the implementation of the program. Such feedback may be built into the design, with clear provision for sequential analysis of the results. In other cases, however, the evaluator must use considerable restraint in order not to "contaminate" the intervention with premature feedback.

Finally, the last four stages of the program evaluation model shown in Fig. 10 require discussion. In the fifth through seventh stages, the results of the program, both in its implementation and its outcome, are analyzed and reported. In the final stage—social policy analysis—the health program evaluator draws out "the best or most useful findings" and presents them in such a way to be useful to program administrators, policy decision-makers, and the health field at large. These final stages are critical and can also be very demanding. Both the importance and difficulty are related to the dynamic nature of the program, the context within which it was conceived and implemented, and the broader policy issues of interest. In addition, it is at these stages that limitations in the program evaluation design, as well as the accumulated modifications of both the program and its evaluation, become very explicit.

Considering the dynamic nature of the program itself, we might imagine the example of the effectiveness of outreach workers in a neighborhood health center. At the outset, a major concern might have been increasing access to professional services. Outreach workers would be trained to contact families, to assist them in assessing their need for formal health services, to make arrangements for visits to the health center, and then to follow up on these arrangements. The principal goal of the outreach program could be simply stated as increasing the overall number of visits, particularly the number of visits for previously neglected care. Let us assume an evaluation design in which families were randomly assigned to a treatment and control group, with monthly utilization measurements made from records data.

The analysis and reporting of results and the translation of findings into useful information for others who were considering funding or employing outreach services would seem to be straightforward. If the results show the desired effect, this would probably be the case. However, as often happens, we might imagine the situation in which no effect was shown. The first reaction of program personnel would probably be to argue that the utilization measures did not capture the principal intent of the outreach effort. This, in fact, might well be the case, but the experienced evaluator would wish to distinguish among several possibilities: the situation in which the original intent or goals were not adequately specified (and therefore not adequately measured); the situation in which the goals were appropriate to the initial conception of the program, but changed over time; and the situation in which the intervention simply had not achieved its intended objectives.

It is, unfortunately, too often the case that careful consideration of these possibilities becomes of interest to the action team only toward the end of the project rather than at the outset. The health program evaluator should be prepared to assess the merits of these alternatives in developing and interpreting the final report. For example, program dynamics would make it highly likely that outreach workers who set out to assist people in increasing their utilization found that this was not the basic problem faced by the families to whom they were assigned. Thus, a great deal of process activity departing from the original intent may have evolved over the course of the intervention, motivated by an implicit shift in program goals. Careful documentation on an ongoing basis would reveal such a shift. For example, the evaluation measurements might have included outreach worker encounter reports specifying types of problems, types of referrals, and so on. If no evidence in a shift of goals or procedures was evident, data on program implementation, such as turnover rates, could be analyzed. Such an analysis might reveal that families with several outreach workers did not change their behavior, whereas families that had the same outreach worker over the course of the intervention did change. With a high overall turnover rate, this unanticipated facet of the program might have accounted for the absence of an effect, confirming the third explanation and yet putting it in perspective.

Thus, the dynamic nature of the program being evaluated must be considered when writing the final report and communicating the findings to the sponsor and other interested parties. If the intervention or study period is of substantial length, say 2 or more years, changes in the environment will also influence the appropriate focus and content of the policy analysis leading from the results. The degree to which this is the case depends in part on the nature of the particular policy decision-making process associated with the evaluation, as well as on external forces.

In developing the evaluation design, one should at the outset take into consideration the various pressures for and against rapid dissemination of the program, or some version of it, that is being evaluated. That is, some ideas or programs may meet resistance even if the program evaluation demonstrates a strong positive effect. On the other hand, health programs with strong appeal may spread rapidly regardless of the evaluation findings. In instances of slow dissemination, the major emphasis of the report would be on the overall merit of the idea or program; in instances of rapid dissemination, more attention would need to be paid to the relationships between various levels of goals and the particular circumstances under which the intervention was most and least successful.

For example, before the evaluation of the Experimental Medical Care Review Organizations (EMCRO) sponsored by the National Center for Health Services Research and Development could be completed, Congress had passed, and The Department of Health, Education and Welfare was in the process of implementing, Professional Standards Review Organizations (PSRO), a closely related concept. The most valuable information to be derived from the EMCRO projects, at least in the intermediate run, had to do with immediate performance and intermediate objectives, rather than ultimate objectives. That is, the decision on disseminating the idea of quality review in the form of PSROs was not dependent on the demonstration of effectiveness by the EMCRO experiments. At the same time, much that had been learned in the EMCRO experience could be transferred to the PSRO implementation process. In a similar example, the use of coronary care units for the treatment of ischemic heart disease is a widely diffused innovation. Nevertheless, Mathers' randomized clinical trial comparing treatment in the CCU with treatment at home, which raised very serious questions about the efficacy of the CCU, has served the useful purpose of greatly increasing interest in assessing the merits of various lengths of stay and the circumstances under which treatment in the CCU may be valuable.[9]

Thus, the interpretation of health program evaluation results depends on the social, economic, and technological context prevailing at the time. The focal interests of policy decision-makers seem to change very rapidly, and it is unusual for decisions to await the results of evaluation research. On the other hand, issues surface repeatedly in different guises, and decision-makers do depend on analysis of existing evaluation research findings. The emphasis of an evaluation project's final report may be quite different from that which was conceived at the outset, for the various reasons described above. It is important that the program evaluator not underestimate the time or effort that needs to be devoted to the dissemination of findings in a manner that is useful to the various audiences. Issues concerning the interface between program evaluation and public policy are described in fuller detail in Chapter 6.

Summary

In this chapter, we have discussed a number of issues that arise in the process of implementing health programs, and in implementing the evaluation of such programs. There is a wide range of program settings within which evaluation may take place. These range from complex multi-site social experiments or demonstration programs, to developmental projects and modification of ongoing health programs, to retrospective analysis of natural experiments.

In light of this diversity of settings, a number of organizational issues, of varying complexity, must be considered in health program evaluation. The respective composition of the evaluation team and the action team was described. It was noted that the degree of control that the program evaluator has over the implementation and operation of the program varies from a high level of control in the social experiment to essentially no control in the natural experiment.

In terms of administrative relationships, it was pointed out that, even assuming the most favorable interpersonal relationships, the program evaluation team is bound to be at odds with the action team to some degree from start to finish. This organizational tension arises from a number of factors, including philosophical differences, competition for resources, the burden that evaluation places on the conduct of the program being evaluated, the special role of the program evaluator, and differences in professional values.

After a framework for viewing the evaluation process was given, the problems of program implementation per se were described. We saw that the complexity and time requirements for implementing a new program are typically underestimated. The difficulty need not be the result of opposition or unusual circumstances, but rather can arise simply from very ordinary working relationships, inter-agency arrangements, and day-to-day procedures, which accumulate to make even the most seemingly straightforward implementation exceedingly complex. Furthermore, the rewards are limited for persons for whom implementation is a primary responsibility, and, often, inadequate attention is paid to clear-cut management responsibility. Implementation is hindered, particularly when multiple organizations are involved. This is true in part because of different perceptions of goals and objectives but also because of uneven interests in program implementation and its coordination.

In the final section, the synchronization of program implementation and program evaluation implementation was discussed. A major issue arises early in the process as the evaluator seeks to obtain clear specification of program goals. It was pointed out that, because of the dynamic nature of programs, multiple goals and measures are desirable. In addition, caution was expressed about trying to settle on measurable goals prematurely. It was suggested that encouraging the action team to focus on the larger objectives of the program rather than on their own performance would allay many fears that arise.

The important issue of delays in both program implementation and the implementation of the evaluation was considered, in addition to the inevitable difficulty of program drift. Several suggestions were offered for dealing with this problem.

Finally, the assessment of outcomes and the reporting of results were discussed. Because of the dynamic nature of both the program and its environment, it was stressed that the health program evaluator needs to be prepared to describe accurately the program as it was actually conducted, rule out alternative explanations for the results obtained, and place these results in the context of current public policy interest. Reporting of program results should take into account whether the program is likely to be rapidly or slowly disseminated, as well as the changing interest of policy decision-makers. The broader issue of the relationship between the evaluation and policy formulation will be considered next, in Chapter 6.

References

1. Andrew, G.: Some observations on management problems in applied social research, Am. Sociol. May, 1967, pp. 85, 86, 87.
2. Mechanic, D.: Evaluation in alcohol, drug abuse, and mental health programs: problems and prospects. In Zusman, J., and Wurster, C. R., editors: Program evaluation: alcohol, drug abuse, and mental health services, Lexington, Mass., 1975, Lexington Books, pp. 5, 21.
3. Riecken, H. W., and Boruch, R. F.: Social experimentation: a method for planning and evaluating social intervention, New York, 1974, Academic Press, Inc., pp. 160, 162.
4. D'Costa, A., and Sechrest, L.: Program evaluation concepts for health administrators, Washington, D.C., 1976, Association of University Programs in Health Administration, pp. 21, 22.
5. Williams, W., and Elmore, R. F., editors: Social program implementation, New York, 1976, Academic Press, Inc., pp. 20, 23.
6. Elinson, J., and Herr, C. E. A.: A sociomedical view of neighborhood health centers, Medical Care 8:97-103, 1970.
7. Pressman, J. L., and Wildavsky, A. B.: Implementation, Berkeley, 1973, University of California Press, pp. 93-94, 97.
8. Weiss, C. H.: Evaluation research: methods of assessing program effectiveness, Englewood Cliffs, N.J., 1972, Prentice-Hall, Inc., pp. 28, 98.
9. Cochrane, A. L.: Effectiveness and efficiency: random reflections on health services, London, 1972, Nuffield Provincial Hospitals Trust, Oxford University Press, pp. 50-54.

Suggested readings

Andrew, G.: Some observations on management problems in applied social research, Am. Sociol. May, 1967, pp. 84-92.

Cochrane, A. L.: Effectiveness and efficiency: random reflections on health services, London, 1972, Nuffield Provincial Hospitals Trust, Oxford University Press.

Pressman, J. L., and Wildavsky, A. B.: Implementation, Berkeley, 1973, University of California Press.

Riecken, H. W., and Boruch, R. F.: Social experimentation: a method for planning and evaluating social intervention, New York, 1974, Academic Press, Inc.

Weikel, K., Yordy, K. D., Goldman, L., Beasley, J. D., and Ellis, E. F.: Evaluation of national health programs, Am. J. Public Health **61:**1801-1831, 1971.

Weiss, C. H.: Evaluation research: methods of assessing program effectiveness, Englewood Cliffs, N.J., 1972, Prentice-Hall, Inc.

Williams, W., and Elmore, R. F., editors: Social program implementation, New York, 1976, Academic Press, Inc.

Zusman, J., and Wurster, C. R., editors: Program evaluation: alcohol, drug abuse, and mental health services, Lexington, Mass., 1975, Lexington Books.

CHAPTER 6

Future issues: evaluation research and public policy

In Chapter 1, a number of reasons were given for the current growth in evaluation research. Prominent among these were an increased demand for accountability by the American public, the increased growth in health services financed or directly provided by the federal government, and the continued growth of new technology. These factors, plus many of the others discussed in Chapter 1, raise several issues concerning the relationship between evaluation research and the development of public policy in health care.

At first glance, these issues appear far removed from the daily experiences of administrators, providers, and planners. But issues such as national health insurance, reimbursement of health care facilities, control of capital expenditures, and a variety of related regulatory concerns will have, and are currently having, a direct impact on the daily operations of health care delivery organizations. For example, a recent evaluation of the Sacramento Medical Care Foundation Certified Hospital Admission Program (CHAP),[1] a precursor of Professional Standards Review Organizations (PSROs), has recently been criticized for a number of flaws in its evaluation design.[2] As the critique notes: "Significant deficiencies in evaluating its impact may mean that the success of CHAP has not been demonstrated and, hence, that an adequate basis for formulating certain national peer review policies may not exist."[2]

It is therefore important for administrators, planners, and providers to understand some of the problems involved in the uses of evaluation research in the development of public policy. This chapter will provide a brief introduction to some of these issues and will suggest some strategies for improving the usefulness of health program evaluation findings to those involved in policy formulation. Some suggestions and predictions for the future growth of evaluation research are also presented.

Current problems in the use of evaluation research to develop public policy

Lumsdaine and Bennett have observed that science is primarily concerned with moving from facts to *understanding*, while program evaluation is primarily concerned with proceeding from facts to *decisions*.[3] Several observers, however, have criticized the relative ineffectiveness of health services program evaluation in contributing to useful decisions, particularly in the development of public policy.[4-6] The problem is not unique to health services. For example, a recent study conducted by Caplan and others of the use of social science knowledge in national policy decisions revealed particular problems with regard to (1) the quality of program evaluations undertaken, (2) the ability to anticipate politically important events and issues, (3) the naïveté of the social scientist concerning political decision-making, and (4) mutual mistrust between the researcher and the decision-maker.[7]

Several of the issues suggested by Caplan's findings have been developed in a systematic fashion by Coleman, who makes a distinction between "decision-oriented" and "conclusion-oriented" research.[8] As implied by the term, decision-oriented research is concerned with the production of information that can be used in the decision-making process by public officials and program creators. In contrast, conclusion-oriented research is primarily concerned with the drawing of inferences that lead to the accumulation of knowledge in the basic disciplines (for example, sociology or economics). These center around issues concerning (1) the timing of information, (2) the redundancy of information, (3) classes of variables, (4) formulation of problems, and (5) dissemination of program findings. Each of these is briefly discussed in the following paragraphs.

Timing of information

Policy-makers operate in a world of immediacy. They have a high need for current information, judgment, and opinion and cannot afford to wait until "all the results are in." This is in contrast to discipline-based academic research, where emphasis is given to refinement and validation of models, and waiting until "all the evidence is in." For policy-makers, timely information based on only partial results is better than completely validated information, which may only be available after it has outlived its usefulness to the decision-maker. Thus, in the design of a program evaluation, one should provide a number of intervening data collection periods, at which point the program can be assessed in a preliminary fashion and the results communicated to decision-makers. This, of course, runs the risk that early results may prove to be wrong. This is particularly the case if a markedly new program is being introduced and is not expected to be stabilized for several months or years. Results based on the first few months of operation may not be the same as those that occur after the program has existed for several years. Consequently, public decision-makers may be wrong in encouraging widespread use of such a program, basing their decision on early results. The trade-off between early release of information and stability of early findings must be assessed. However, in major social programs, this may be less of a problem, since it generally takes several years for such programs to be passed either by the legislative or by the executive branch of government. Thus, early results can be given to policy-makers while time is made available to await final results. By keeping in close touch with policy-makers, program evaluators can maintain a type of ongoing dialogue which facilitates the refinement of program findings as they occur.

Redundancy of information

Related to the idea of timely, though incomplete, results is the notion of redundancy of information. Unlike academic research in which parsimony of theory is desirable, policy research thrives on multiple assumptions. A policy-maker needs to know the pros and cons of a number of alternative courses of action. Thus, multiple sources of data and methods of data analysis are useful. In this way, policy-makers and their staff can check on the validity of information and draw inferences from different findings that may rest on different assumptions.

Classes of variables

Policy research must generally work with *three* classes of variables (policy outcome variables, policy variables, and situational variables), while academic research typically is concerned with only two main classes of variables—independent variables and dependent variables. In policy research, while the dependent variables are policy outcomes, the independent variables must be separated into two classes: one class of variables that can be manipulated by public policy and a second class of "situational" variables that cannot be manipulated by public policy. For example, the Rand Health Insurance Experiment[9] is intended to assess the impact of different mechanisms of financial coverage for medical services on patient utilization of those services (situational variables) and also the impact of various forms of insurance coverage with different co-insurance and deductible options. These latter variables, that is, the co-insurance and deductibles, constitute the policy manipulable variables, while patient characteristics such as age, sex, and race constitute that cannot be directly manipulated by public policy. From a policy perspective, the primary variables of interest are obviously those that can be directly affected by public policy. Variables that cannot be manipulated are of less interest, although not unimportant. For example, they do help to identify certain target groups in the population for whom the particular change in public policy may have differential effects. Nevertheless, it is important to keep these two sets of variables distinct.

Formulation of problems

In policy research, the problem comes from outside the academic discipline and must be carefully translated into the research setting without loss of its operational significance. This is in contrast to academic research, which usually begins with the researcher formulating a question or problem to be addressed. For the researcher, this frequently involves a controversy over competing theories or explanations of a particular phenomenon. But in the world of the decision-maker, problems do not come neatly categorized as "sociological," "economic," or "psychological," but rather as specific issues that need to be addressed and frequently cut across various academic disciplines. Thus, the potential usefulness of policy research depends critically on understanding the problem as defined by decision-makers and specifying the various subcomponents of the problem in terms of its public policy implications rather than its implications for developing a particular disciplinary theory.

Dissemination of findings

Finally, there is the need to present results in a way that can be understood by those in decision-making positions. While academic research is frequently disseminated in scientific journals for the purpose of communicating with one's colleagues in a particular discipline, policy research is intended to result in decision-making changes regarding particular issues and problems. This means using language understandable to the decision-maker, targeting the findings to specific groups interested in them rather than broad-based distribution of results, and, in particular, using face-to-face, verbal reporting. Most public decision-makers do not have time to read 25-page reports, let alone 200-page documents. A more effective strategy is to communicate verbally the highlights of a particular piece of research and then send the written report as background documentation that the decision-maker, or the decision-maker's staff, can examine if necessary. When dealing with legislators and governmental decision-makers, the "10-minute rule" is usually a good maxim to follow. This rule states that anything important must be said in the first 10 minutes, because anything beyond that period is likely to be forgotten.

Summary and "case study"

The preceding discussion describes the basic distinctions between decision-oriented policy research and conclusion-oriented academic research. In policy research, the problems originate from the world of action and the findings are reported back to the world of action. Timely, partial results are to be preferred to complete but outdated findings. Redundancy of information is useful, as is the explicit distinction between variables that can be manipulated by public policy versus those that cannot. Finally, it is important to disseminate results in clear and understandable language to specific groups interested in the problem and to make heavy use of verbal, direct interaction with decision-makers.

While these represent basic distinctions, it is important to emphasize that the actual conduct of policy research does not deviate from academic norms of scientific rigor. The canons of methodology that guide all investigative efforts are equally applicable to policy-oriented program evaluation as they are to academic investigations designed to advance disciplinary knowledge and theory. As was noted in Chapter 5, however, research conducted in live, social action settings does place great strains and demands on the researcher in designing scientifically valid studies while still operating within the constraints of specific political and administrative concerns. In some respects, the importance of a scientifically sound study is more important in program evaluation research than in academic research because the results will be used within a political framework. Critics or detractors of a specific program will be only too happy to punch holes in conclusions opposite to their own by criticizing the methodology and design on which the findings are based. The stronger the design used in a specific program evaluation, the greater the ammunition available to the policy-maker and those concerned with the problem to defend the program's operation, assuming, of course, that the results are basically favorable. Even if the results are not favorable, a strong evaluation may be preferred to a weak one because remedial action may then be taken with greater confidence.

The small effect that current health services research, including specific program evaluation research, has had on public policy may be attributed, at least in part, to the failure of investigators, program administrators, providers, and planners to recognize the principles outlined. Even more persuasive is the recognition that the few successful attempts have generally followed the specific principles outlined above. For example, Myers has described the successful efforts of Dr. Paul Elwood and his Interstudy colleagues in the implementation of the health maintenance organization (HMO) legislation in 1972.[5]

While many health services researchers have felt that the evidence regarding the advantages of prepaid group practice is premature and inconclusive, and that considerable investigative work remains (note the academic perspective), Elwood and colleagues recognized that the *timing* and *climate* of the administration at that time was right for the development of a program based on *partial* and *preliminary* information. They also recognized that the purpose was not to contribute to existing knowledge of prepaid group practice per se, but rather to provide some direct input into social policy which might subsequently be modified by further research results. Further, they recognized that the users or target groups of the research were not other researchers, but rather decision-makers, and thus presented their proposal in a form and manner most useful to decision-makers. This largely involved direct, face-to-face interactions with key government and congressional leaders. They were also particularly sensitive to the policy variables that could be changed versus the situational variables that could not be changed. For example, they broadened the definition of HMOs beyond the notion of simply prepaid group practice, which the majority of physicians reject, to encompass medical care foundation plans and other forms of practice that would make physicians more comfortable with the strategy. They also recognized the situational variable that most consumers are not in prepaid group practice plans and are not likely to enroll in them given the prevailing practice of medicine. They therefore concentrated on the prepayment and cost control aspects of the proposal, rather than suggesting radical restructuring of the health care delivery system.

Based on this "success story" as a departure point, the following section provides some additional ideas on how evaluation research may be more useful to decision-makers in policy-making positions.

Suggestions for improving the use of health program evaluations in the policy-making process

In addition to the comments noted in the preceding section, several structural relationships can facilitate the use of evaluation research results in public decision-making. Drawing on Coleman,[10] Andersen has developed five propositions specific to health services program evaluation that, if validated, would provide useful guidelines for more effective efforts.[4] These are briefly outlined here.

1. The greater the lateral distance between the problem-formulator and the decision-maker, the less likely it is that questions relevant to the decision-maker will be researched, and, hence, research results utilized.

This means that private foundations, independent research groups, and university-based research groups trying to formulate research questions of relevance to legislators and practitioners are likely to experience difficulty. The formulators of the problem and the decision-makers are members of different organizations, with widely varying perspectives, and likely to have limited communication with each other. As a result, there is likely to be an incongruence and misperception of the dimensions of the research and the uses to which it might be put.

As previously indicated, it is important to identify those in need of the information and let those groups delineate the administrative and political dimensions of the problem. They should also be involved in discussions of the types of data to be collected. This enables them to have some advance understanding of how the data are related to the specific problem at hand and, thereby, assists them in making more rapid use of the eventual program findings.[11]

Furthermore, since it is unrealistic to expect most decision-makers to be thoroughly familiar with the methodological tools of evaluation researchers, it may be helpful to have individuals who can act as "technical brokers" to the decision-makers.[11] These would be individuals who can translate the program results and methodologies into terms that are understandable to the policy-maker. It is important that such communication take place on a continuous basis so that there is constant interplay between the evaluation researcher, the broker, and the decision-maker. Such feedback will help to ensure that the program findings continue to be relevant to the decision-maker. The decision-maker, in turn, can communicate to the evaluator sudden changes in political climate that may require that the evaluation focus more on certain objectives than on others.

2. Research results are more likely to be utilized if the problem-formulator has status and authority equal to or greater than that of the decision-maker.

The validity of this proposition is perhaps best indicated by the number of demonstration projects frequently undertaken by operating departments in organizations, which seldom succeed because they must really be implemented and supported by higher administrative officials within the organizations. For example, the results of a hospital medical audit program are not likely to be used unless physician leaders, hospital administrators, and the board of trustees see the importance of the findings and have been involved in formulating the issues addressed by the audit.

3. Research is more likely to be implemented if the policy-formulator considered all interested groups than if the formulator considered only some of these groups in a dispersed authority decision structure.

For example, evaluations that may be conducted by the health systems agencies are more likely to be accepted and utilized if they have taken into account all relevant groups, including providers, consumers, and other regulatory agencies.

4. The less the organizational autonomy of the researcher from those who use the results or those who formulate the problem, the less likely the research will deal with other than the immediate concerns of the organization.

Close involvement of the researcher with the funder and user of the results may lead to questions that are relevant but too narrowly focused. Thus, evaluation of new forms of delivering medical care by a group that is being funded by the sponsor of the innovation may result in findings that are of some pertinence but may ignore other considerations that might have been elicited by an outside evaluation group funded from separate sources. In brief, the results may be unduly narrow and therefore less likely to be used by decision-makers.

5. The closer the research to a third party who is not the problem-formulator or decision-maker, the greater the probability that the research result will be irrelevant to policy decisions and therefore not utilized.

This, of course, is opposite to the proposition suggested just before. Evaluations conducted by completely autonomous researchers may address issues that might be of interest in building a theory of health services delivery but may ignore or downplay those items of direct interest to the agency involved with the program. Inevitably, there are trade-offs concerning the relative autonomy of evaluation research vis-a-vis its potential use to decision-makers. High autonomy of the evaluation research unit may lead to comprehensiveness of findings but lack of focus, while little autonomy may lead to immediate program relevancy but a narrow perspective. Both situations can result in less useful information that is less likely to be used by decision-makers. The trick, of course, is to find an accommodation along the continuum of autonomy that will be most compatible with the objectives of the decision-maker and the potential usefulness and utility of the findings.

In addition to these "structural" suggestions, three other factors can contribute to a greater use of program evaluation results in public policy decision-making. These include (1) the provision of long-term trend information, (2) the development of a "standby research capability," and (3) the development of more coherent theories of how health services programs operate.

The development of long-range policies in health delivery is one of the most difficult problems facing health services decision-makers. Program evaluators can assist in this effort by making more judicious use of secondary analysis of existing data as well as by developing well-designed longitudinal studies. Data from such analyses can provide information of long-run value to decision-makers. Examples include ongoing work in the development of health status indices, measures of access to health services, and the longitudinal assessment of such interventions as that suggested by the Rand Health Insurance Experiment.[9]

It would also be mutually beneficial if federal government officials and the health services community could work cooperatively in developing an information network for keeping track of natural experiments and attempt to assess them as they occur. Klarman has noted that natural experiments have a primary advantage over demonstration projects because the latter usually take place under artificially favorable conditions in which the program results are not likely to hold when generalized to other situations.[12] The ability to assess natural experiments also depends crucially on what Biderman terms "standby research capability."[13] In brief, it is necessary to have long-term baseline data on various aspects of health care delivery in order to take advantage of naturally occurring experiments from which the "post" data can be collected.

Fortunately, various standby research capabilities are being increased through a more systematic collection of data on health system variables. Examples include the continued work of the National Center for Health Statistics, including the development of a National Ambulatory Medical Care Survey;[14] the studies of health services use conducted by the Center for Health Administration Studies, and the National Opinion Research Center, University of Chicago;[15,16] the information that will be derived from the Rand Health Insurance Experiment;[9] and a study being conducted by the National Center for Health Services Research concerned with medical care expenditures.[17] All of these data provide, or will provide, useful baseline measures for assessing future interventions, be they planned or unplanned. Examples include outbreaks in various diseases, sudden changes in program financing, and future reorganization of health services.

Finally, one must recognize the continuing need for better theory to support health services program evaluation and to help increase the use of program evaluation results in public decision-making. It may seem that such a suggestion runs counter to much of what has been said in preceding sections, but an important distinction must be made between the relevance of theory to increase use of health program evaluation (theory as a means to an end) and the conduct of research exclusively to increase theoretical knowledge (as an end in itself). Coleman notes that theory as an end is not the purpose of evaluation research, and studies whose primary purpose is to develop further theory are likely to be less useful and less used by decision-makers. In contrast, however, there is a great need in public policy-making in health care for the use of theory as a means to more effective decision-making. Little is currently known about the interrelationships among the various parts of the health care delivery system, and, therefore, it is not possible to construct an overall health policy or agenda for health policy, even if one ignores the political and other constraints on the development of such a policy.

As Zucker[18] has noted in relation to social problems in general, there is a great lack of cumulative knowledge in evaluation research of health services because of reliance on a piece-by-piece or problem-by-problem approach. In essence, each problem is treated as unique. Alcoholism is studied as alcoholism, hypertension compliance is treated as hypertension compliance, cost-control problems are treated as cost-control problems. As a result, relationships between these problems are not conceptualized, are not taken into account in evaluative designs, and thus provide no basis for constructing consolidated theory from which program interdependencies may be considered in the development of public policy. The fact that the assessment of alcoholism treatment programs may share many common elements with the assessment of hypertension compliance programs is generally not considered. In turn, the relationship between (1) the issues of utilization and compliance in alcoholism treatment and in hypertension compliance programs in reference to the cost of medical care and (2) strategies for controlling cost regarding patient/provider behavior is ignored.

The need to consider the more general properties of health program evaluation is also indicated by the extent to which problems come into vogue and then fade away. Cohen has identified the "half-life" of a social problem as approximately 3 years.[18] The half-life of health services issues would appear to be about the same length, as evidenced by the varying concerns and attention given in recent years to mental health, alcoholism and drug addiction, long-term care, and, most recently, self-care.

If evaluations are designed to focus on specific problems, which fade away and come back again, it is not possible to build cumulative knowledge that can be translated into the public policy-making process on a broader level. What is needed is the development of theoretical frameworks that will guide evaluations of different health services problems. In many cases, exploratory rather than experimental or quasi-experimental evaluations may prove more useful for generating such frameworks. In other cases, greater attention should be given to basic social science theory that already exists and can be used by program evaluators to assist administrators and policy-makers in understanding the phenomenon under study. In the end, only the building of cumulative knowledge of the health care delivery process will provide long-run guidance for people operating at policy-making positions within various levels of government.

All of the above suggestions and comments depend on the cooperation and collaboration of evaluation researchers, program administrators, providers, planners, and those in policy-making positions. As May notes:

> Important opportunities for innovation, improvement and refinement of the health services delivery system are lost because of the administrators' lack of awareness of research findings or their inability to use them. At the same time much time and money is being invested in research that addresses questions not relevant to current needs of decision-makers or is too abstract or narrowly oriented to be useful to them. Research and development are too important to leave the research design and execution responsibility solely to the researchers. And it is too important to leave the choice of questions and their formulation to administrators. The focus, content, quality, pertinence, and timeliness of health services research efforts represent areas for which all interested parties share responsibility.[19]

Future directions

As indicated at several points in this text, program evaluation research in health services is likely to grow in future years. Assumptions about many health program innovations are largely untested. Programs thought to work well in theory or in isolated settings frequently fail to hold up in daily practice. For example, a recent review of twenty-eight social and medical innovations revealed that only 20 percent of the programs were judged to be "quite successful," another 20 percent were judged to have resulted in "some success," while the remaining 60 percent were judged to have either no positive effect or even a harmful effect.[20]

Given this fact, society will demand that those involved in the delivery of health services learn more about themselves and the programs for which they are responsible, however painful this process might be. This assessment will take two primary forms. The first will follow Campbell's notion of the "experimenting society"[21] based on the experimental method. The second, however, will be based on the growth of process-oriented evaluation concerned with understanding how particular programs are intended to operate and assessing the extent to which they have been implemented. The choice between the two basic procedures will likely depend on many factors, but a key determinant is likely to be the degree of knowledge of the phenomenon under study. The more that is known about how a particular program operates and the theory behind it, the more possible and logical it becomes to evaluate the program in an experimental or quasi-experimental fashion. The less that is known about a program, the more it makes sense to simply try to understand the basic components of the program and the degree to which it is ever possible to implement it.

A somewhat different way of viewing the above issue is in terms of the degree of certainty of one's beliefs concerning the cause-and-effect relationships involved in the program and the degree of certainty regarding preferences for possible outcomes. These two dimensions are used by Thompson in the development of a typology of decision strategies for organizations.[22] They are also useful, however, for considering various forms of program evaluation, as shown in Table 12.

In Table 12, *computational* decisions exist when both beliefs about cause/effect relationships and preferences regarding the desirability of outcomes are certain. In such cases there is little need for formal program evaluation, although ongoing monitoring may be necessary. Childhood immuniza-

Table 12. Decision-making factors affecting the choice of future program evaluations

Beliefs about cause/effect relationships	*Preferences regarding desirability of possible outcomes*	
	Certain	*Uncertain*
Certain	*Computational* No need for formal program evaluation efforts, although ongoing monitoring is important	*Compromise* Rigorous program evaluation efforts useful in selling and defending the program in political battles, particularly if program effects are small
Uncertain	*Judgmental* Impact, summative program evaluation most appropriate	*Inspirational* Process-oriented formative evaluation most appropriate

tion programs represent an example of a basically computational decision where it is known that the vaccine prevents the disease and it is widely agreed that this is a preferable outcome. In such cases, only ongoing monitoring of effort, in terms of levels of immunization, is needed.

As shown in the upper right-hand cell of Table 12, *compromise* decisions exist where beliefs about cause/effect relationships are certain but there is little agreement regarding the desirability of various outcomes. This situation is perhaps best illustrated by the fluoridation of public water supplies. There exists general agreement that fluoridated water will result in fewer dental caries, but in some communities disagreement exists (however irrational it may seem to public health professionals) regarding the relative desirability of this outcome versus fear of contaminated water supplies and invasion of personal rights. In such cases, rigorous experimental evaluations can be useful as a defense against critics who will attempt to refute the scientific evidence by criticizing the study design, methodology, and analysis. This is particularly true when the alleged beneficial effects of the program are small to moderate.

The lower left-hand cell of Table 12 indicates *judgmental* decisions in which beliefs about cause/effect relationships are uncertain but consensus exists concerning the desirability of certain outcomes. It is in this area that the majority of impact program evaluations will take place. The evaluation of quality assurance programs serves as an example. There exists considerable uncertainty regarding the actual effect of such programs on the quality of medical care, yet wide consensus that improved quality of care is a desirable outcome (although not necessarily at *any* cost).

Finally, the lower right-hand cell of Table 12 shows the existence of *inspirational* judgments in which there is little agreement on cause/effect relationships and little consensus on the desirability of outcomes. It is perhaps illustrated by the development of self-care programs. Beliefs about the cause/effect relationships of such activities are not thoroughly documented at present, nor is there widespread agreement regarding the possible desirability of various outcomes of having consumers treat themselves. In such programs, it makes the most sense to simply try to clearly define the specifics of self-care activities, see to what extent they are accurately followed in various demonstration programs, and then, after the basic process of various programs has been described, go on to try to document program impact over a long period of time.

Roos notes it will be increasingly important in future years to fit program evaluation research strategies to the specific nature of the program under study and the types of decisions to be made.[23] Programs with clearly defined goals and objectives, where it is possible to obtain a high degree of knowledge, are appropriate for experimental and quasi-experimental designs. In contrast, programs that have ill-defined goals, that are in their beginning stages, and that show a low degree of obtainable knowledge are more appropriate for process-oriented formative evaluations.

The preceding factors influencing future direction and growth of evaluation research are, of course, oversimplified. Numerous other factors, again many of them already mentioned in Chapter 1, will influence the direction and growth of health services program evaluations. Nevertheless, three certainties do emerge. The first is that program evaluations of both a process-oriented and an impact-oriented nature will continue to grow, for the reasons cited above and in Chapter 1. Second, program administrators, providers, planners, evaluation researchers, and policy-makers will need to become increasingly sophisticated about the problems and issues involved in assessing health care programs. This ranges all the way from being better able to specify program objectives, components, and categories of evaluation, to the consideration of alternative research designs, data collection strategies, assessment of the reliability and validity of measures, appropriate choice of data analysis, and increased competence in making sure that the results of the program evaluation effort are useful to and used by the decision-makers for whom they are intended.

The third certainty follows from the first two: namely, that there will be an increased need for training health professionals of all categories and exposing them to some of the basic considerations involved in the evaluation of health care programs. Health care professionals will need to have a common understanding of the basic issues in assessing programs and be able to speak a common language. A thorough understanding of the issues raised in this book will provide a starting point toward this objective. It will in no way substitute for the experience of daily professional practice, but it will help those involved to interpret, integrate, and learn from such experiences. In the process of engaging in program evaluation activities, health professionals may also learn more about themselves, in addition to their program. Such self-discovery can contribute to increased personal and professional growth.

References

1. Brian, E.: Government control of hospital utilization: a California experience, N. Engl. J. Med. **286:**1342, 1972.
2. Sayetta, R. B.: Critique of an earlier study of the Sacramento Medical Care Foundation Certified Hospital Admission Program (CHAP), Medical Care **14:**80-90, 1976.
3. Lumsdaine, A. A., and Bennett, C. A.: Assessing alternative conceptions of evaluation. In Bennett, C. A., and Lumsdaine, A. A., editors: Evaluation and experiment, New York, 1975, Academic Press, Inc., p. 538.
4. Andersen, R.: Social factors influencing administrators' use of research results—some hypotheses, Inquiry **12:**235-258, 1975.
5. Myers, B. A.: Health services research and health policy: interactions, Medical Care **11:**352-358, 1973.
6. Williams, S., and Wysong, J.: The uses of research and national health policy: an assessment and agenda, Medical Care **13:**256-267, 1975.
7. Caplan, N., Morrison, A., and Stambaugh, R. J.; The use of social science knowledge in policy decisions at the national level, Ann Arbor, 1975, Institute for Social Research, University of Michigan.
8. Coleman, J.: Policy research in social sciences, Morristown, N. J., 1972, General Learning Press, pp. 1-23.
9. Newhouse, J. P.: A design for a health insurance experiment, Inquiry **11:**5-27, 1974.
10. Coleman, J. S.: The social structure surrounding policy research, Chicago, 1974, University of Chicago.
11. Rich, R. F.: Selective utilization of social science related information by federal policy makers, Inquiry **12:**39-245, 1975.
12. Klarman, H.: National health policies and planning for health services, Milbank Memorial Fund Quarterly **54:**1-28, 1976.
13. Biderman, A. D.: Anticipatory studies and stand-by research capabilities. In Bauer, R. A., editor: Social indicators, Cambridge, Mass., 1966, The M.I.T. Press, pp. 272-301.
14. National Center for Health Statistics: National ambulatory medical care statistics: background and methodology, Vital and health statistics, Series 2, No. 61, DHEW

Publication No. (HRA)74-1335, Washington, D.C., 1974, U.S. Government Printing Office.

15. Andersen, R., Kravits, J., and Anderson, O. W.: Equity in health services: empirical analysis and social policy, Cambridge, Mass., 1975, Ballinger Publishing Co.

16. Anderson, R., Lions, J., and Anderson, O. W.: Two decades of health services, Chicago, 1976, University of Chicago Press.

17. Walden, D.: National medical care expenditures survey, National Center for Health Services Research and National Center for Health Statistics (in press).

18. Zucker, L.: Evaluating evaluation research: what are the standards for judging research quality? Sociol. Pract. **2:**107-124, Fall 1977.

19. May, J. J.: Symposium: the policy uses of research—introduction, Inquiry **12:**230, 1975.

20. Gilbert, J. P., Light, R. P., and Mosteller, F.: Assessing social innovations: an empirical base for policy. In Bennett, C. A., and Lumsdaine, A. A., editors: Evaluation and experiment, New York, 1975, Academic Press, Inc., pp. 113-114.

21. Campbell, D. T.: Reforms as experiments, Am. Psychol. **24:**409-429, 1969.

22. Thompson, J. D.: Organizations in action, New York, 1967, McGraw-Hill Book Co.

23. Roos, N. P.: Evaluation, quasi-experimentation, and public policy: observations by a short-term bureaucrat. In Caporaso, J., and Roos, L. L., Jr., editors: Quasi-experiments: testing theory and evaluating policy, Chicago, 1973, Northwestern University Press.

Suggested readings

Caplan, N., Morrison, A., and Stambaugh, R. J.: The use of social science knowledge in policy decisions at the national level, Ann Arbor, 1975, Institute for Social Research, University of Michigan.

Coleman, J.: Policy research in social sciences, Morristown, N.J., 1972, General Learning Press, pp. 1-23.

Myers, B. A.: Health services research and health policy: interactions, Medical Care **11:**352-358, 1973.

Symposium: the policy uses of research, Inquiry **12:**228-262, 1975.

Weikel, K.: Evaluation of national health programs: a departmental view, Am. J. Public Health **61:**1801-1802, 1971.

Williams, S., and Wysong, J.: The uses of research and national health policy: an assessment and agenda, Medical Care **13:**256-267, 1975.

Williams, W., and Elmore, R.: Social program implementation, New York, 1976, Academic Press, Inc.

Yordy, K. D.: Evaluation of national health programs: on the federal level, Am. J. Public Health **61:**1803-1808, 1971.

Multiple time series evaluation of a cervical cancer screening program

Sharon Baker

Statement of the problem

The tool for early detection of cervical cancer, the Pap test, has been available since before World War II. This test has been demonstrated to be inexpensive, acceptable to most women, and highly reliable. When detected early, cervical cancer is very susceptible to cure without producing the psychological and physical disability that follows the treatment of breast cancer, for example.

In spite of these facts, cervical cancer still accounts for a high proportion of cancer deaths. It is the fourth most common cause of death for white women ages 40 to 45 and for black women 35 to 40. In Washington state, about 135 women die each year from cervical cancer.

Efforts by the American Cancer Society and the health professions to educate women to the importance of regular Pap testing have been encouragingly successful with middle and upper socioeconomic women. Younger women from these groups are particularly conscientious about Pap testing. Unfortunately, these educational efforts have been least effective with women who, on the basis of epidemiological data, are at exaggerated risk for cervical cancer, that is, older women, particularly women from lower socioeconomic groups. Various factors prevent these women from obtaining regular Pap testing. They include financial and educational barriers, cultural patterns, and the pressures of daily living. High percentages of women at exaggerated risk for cervical cancer *have not been motivated by conventional health education methods.* In funding the cervical cancer screening program for Washington state, the National Cancer Institute is seeking models which will facilitate the screening of these high-risk populations.

The model for addressing the problem
Program objectives

Objectives of the funding agency. In issuing the request for proposal for the implementation of a cervical cancer screening program, the National Cancer Institute outlined the following objectives:

1. To reduce the incidence of, and mortality from, invasive cancer of the cervix uteri through cytologic examinations among high-risk women
2. To provide funds to the nation's state and territorial health departments to supplement, expand, or initiate ongoing programs for cervical cancer screening
3. To encourage state health departments to develop cervical cancer screening programs in close coordination with other state agencies, federal agencies, and appropriate private agencies

4. To encourage the use of high quality pathology laboratory procedures by qualified personnel
5. To develop a system by which women are screened yearly by a Pap test
6. To encourage cervical screening activites that will assure appropriate medical management for all high-risk women with positive or suspicious Pap test results
7. To identify and employ those factors that optimize the cost-effectiveness of cervical cancer screening programs using the Pap test
8. To develop, assemble, and provide to the cervical cancer screening program systematic data on the evaluations of state cervical cancer screening programs

Objectives of the Washington State Cervical Cancer Screening Program. The objectives of the program are as follows:

1. To screen 30 percent of the defined target population in the first year, 60 percent in the second year, and 80 percent in the third year of the program
2. To assure follow-up and the establishment of a definitive diagnosis for women with atypical Pap results
3. To assure diagnosis, treatment, and rehabilitation for cervical cancer that are up to standards established by the advisory board
4. To compute the unit costs per screening, per case brought to diagnosis, and per case brought to treatment on a yearly basis
5. To evaluate the effect of removing financial barriers to screening for high-risk populations

This proposed evaluation will focus primarily on objectives *a* and *e,* that is, the extent to which the program really does result in an increase in the number of women receiving Pap smears.

Assumptions underlying program objectives

1. Morbidity and mortality from cervical cancer can be reduced by screening programs.

The strongest evidence for this assumption comes from a review of existing screening programs. In British Columbia a cervical screening program has been promoted for over 20 years. Each year increasing percentages of the population are screened. Mortality rates for cervical cancer in British Columbia were 11.4 per 100,000 in 1958. By 1973 the rate had dropped to 5.6 per 100,000.[1, 2] A comparison of these rates to the rates in other parts of Canada without a vigorous screening program revealed that the mortality rates in British Columbia were significantly lower than those in other provinces.[3]

Stage at treatment is a critical factor in morbidity and mortality from cervical cancer. The American Cancer Society[4] suggests that 5-year survival rates for localized cervical cancer are 82 percent but drop to 44 percent for tumors with regional involvement. Screening programs in Norway[5] and Finland[6] have been successful in improving the stage distribution for invasive cervical cancer in those countries.

2. Screening programs directed at populations at exaggerated risk for cervical cancer are likely to be more cost-effective than nondirected screening.

Reported morbidity and mortality rates for cervical cancer are often difficult to analyze because of wide disparities in rates between various populations. Four factors in particular are associated with exaggerated risk for cervical cancer.[7] These factors are age, race, socioeconomic status, and marital and sexual factors.

Age. Both morbidity and mortality for cervical cancer increase with increasing age. However, the disease has its greatest impact on mortality in white women ages 40 to 44 and black women ages 35 to 39. In those age groups it is the fourth leading cause of death.[8]

Race. Mortality from cervical cancer not only occurs earlier in black women, but it has been demonstrated that the incidence of the disease is about twice as high in black women as in white women.[4] Repeated studies have verified a lower rate of cervical cancer in Jewish women than in any other race.[7] Rates for American Indian, Chicano, and Asian American women have not been as thoroughly investigated.

Socioeconomic status. A number of studies have verified an inverse relationship between socioeconomic status and risk for cervical cancer.[7] This relationship is probably related to differential utilization of Pap smears between socioeconomic groups,[9] and to varying cultural patterns in sexual and marital relationships.

Marital and sexual factors. A clear relationship exists between heterosexual activity and risk for cervical cancer.[10] Increased risk is associated with early age at first coitus and multiple sexual partners. The underlying etiological factors in this relationship have not yet been identified but are probably associated with exposure to certain infections or other potentially carcinogenic agents such as male smegma[11] or sperm.[12]

In attempts to develop models for evaluating the cost-effectiveness of screening for disease, cervical cancer is frequently taken as the prime example of disease in which screening is likely to be cost-effective.[13, 14] This is particularly the case since screening efforts can be directed at populations at exaggerated risk which can be identified on the basis of demographic information such as age and socioeconomic status.

Method for reaching these objectives

Seven Washington counties were chosen in which to focus the implementation of this program. They were chosen on the basis of demographic data which reflects risk for cervical cancer, such as high percentages of low-income and minority women. In addition, existing health care delivery facilities and community support for the program were also considered in selection.

The target population is defined as:

Women over 16 (special emphasis will be given to recruiting women over 40 for screening)

Who have family incomes at or below 200% of HEW poverty guidelines (currently, this is about $9,000 a year for a family of four)

Who have not had a Pap smear in the last year, or who have a medical indication for a Pap smear

Education and *motivation* of the target population will be the responsibility of the county units of the American Cancer Society Uterine Task Force working in cooperation with local groups who represent the target population. These local groups have been working together throughout the planning phase.

Clinical screening is provided in existing health facilities including physicans' offices, family planning clinics, and community clinics. Minimum standards for the screening examination include:

A gynecological history

Breast examination

Pap smear

Bimanual examination

Clinics and individuals providing the service are compensated on the basis of the number of patients from the target population screened. The fee ($12 per screenee) is based on an analysis of the cost of providing care and on the basis of recommendations from the advisory board of health professionals. Providers of screening services will be expected to complete a Unit Screening Report on each patient screened. Funding will also be available for diagnostic tests needed to establish a definitive diagnosis such as colposcopy, cervical biopsy, or conization. Under NCI guidelines, no funding is available for treatment.

Cytologic specimens will be sent to the laboratory chosen by the screening facility that meets minimum standards to ensure quality screening for less than $3 per Pap smear. A number of regional laboratories have indicated an ability to meet these criteria.

Follow-up and treatment will be ensured by the local screening facility and county public health nurses and will be monitored by the CCSP staff.

The CCSP will be administered through the State Department of Social and Health Services, Adult Health Section.

Questions to be answered in the evaluation

1. Are we reaching and screening the defined target population and achieving necessary follow-up of cases to establish a definitive diagnosis?
2. Are we assuring high-quality screening, treatment, and rehabilitation?
3. What are the unit costs per screening, per case brought to diagnosis, and per case brought to treatment and what proportion of this cost is attributable to administrative and supporting services?
4. Does the CCSP significantly increase the number of Pap smears done in a target county as compared to the number in a matched comparison county?

Methods of evaluation

Sources of data

1. Unit Screening Reports will be completed for each screenee. Information included is year of birth, menopausal status, urban or rural residence, socioeconomic group, race, screening history, examination results, results of further diagnostic measures, and treatment. This information will be available quarterly.

2. Uterine Task Force reports from county units of the ACS outlining educational activities will be available monthly.

3. Maps will be made of each county with socioeconomic rankings of geographic units (primarily CCD) indicating the dispersion of services.

4. Estimates of the level of Pap screening in the selected counties in 1972, 1973, and 1974 will be made. These estimates will also be developed for comparison counties.

Appropriate evaluation designs

Assessment of organizational behavior. The process required to answer the first three evaluation questions posed (Q. 1, 2, 3) is given various labels by evaluators. Suchman[15] would classify the process involved in assessing whether or not the program is reaching, screening, and following up the defined target population (Q. 1) as performance evaluation. Alternatively, this aspect of evaluation could be viewed as adequacy of performance rather than performance because the defined target population is based on an assessment of need for screening among high-risk (low-income) women. Answering the evaluation question on quality of screening, treatment and rehabilitation (Q. 2) would be viewed as a performance evaluation since "need" in this instance is difficult to specify. The evaluation of unit costs per screening and per case (Q. 3) will eventually be part of an efficiency evaluation since NCI is funding a number of programs to assure the screening of high-risk populations throughout the United States. In this way, the unit costs of a variety of models can be compared.

The evaluation of all three of these first questions will also involve a process analysis that will allow program administrators to better make decisions for changes needed to improve program effectiveness.

Williams,[16] on the other hand, would view these activities as intermediate or final implementation analysis; that is, an assessment of whether or not the program was "in place" and functioning in compliance with the original design for achieving the desired objectives. In the case of either classification system, the answers to the first three evaluation questions give information on whether or not the program is doing what it set out to do in terms of organization behavior and do not tell if it is a good thing to do or not. In Williams' terms output will be measured by these means. Outcome or the impact of the program on program participants will not be.

Assessment of program impact. The overriding consideration in a screening program such as this is to reduce the morbidity and mortality associated with cervical cancer. However, several factors prevent the use of cervical cancer morbidity and mortality as an outcome measure in this state. First, Washington is one of many states which do not have a population-based tumor registry for the entire state. Thus, we would be unable to identify a reduction in morbidity and mortality since we do not know what the baseline level is. Data from death certificates are notoriously unreliable in the area of cervical cancer. The second limitation on the use of morbidity and mortality for outcome measures is related to the funding period of the program. Currently NCI is offering funding for a 3-year period. It has been demonstrated in British Columbia[1] that a lag of up to 10 years is required to assess the impact of screening on mortality.

Thus, in lieu of a more direct outcome measure, the evaluation of the impact of the CCSP will be based on an assessment of the level of Pap screening in the seven target counties contrasted to the level in matched comparison counties. The assumption that the level of screening is related to cancer morbidity and mortality was discussed previously.

Design to be employed. A quasi-experimental multiple time-series design will be employed to contrast the level of Pap screening in experimental and matched comparison counties. The variable that will be measured is the ratio between the number of women over 16 in the county and the number of Pap smears reported by laboratories in 1972, 1973, and 1974 prior to the program and in 1975, 1976, 1977, and 1978 during the terms of the program.*

Campbell and Stanley[17] suggest that the multiple time-series design is probably one of the best and most feasible of the quasi-experimental designs. The selection of counties in which to implement the program was made early in the planning primarily on the basis of demographic and vital statistics data indicating higher concentrations of women and exaggerated risk for cervical cancer. Thus, the random assignment of counties to experimental and control groups, a prerequisite for a true experimental design, is not possible. In the absence of a true experimental design, Campbell and Stanley[17] suggest that support for a hypothesis can be increased by the number of "plausible rival hypotheses" or threats to validity which can be controlled for in a quasi-experimental design. The multiple time-series design is able to control for internal sources of invalidity. However, in this application of the design two possible threats to internal validity should be carefully monitored. The first is the effect of history. Subjective reports suggest that after the news of the discovery of breast cancer in two nationally known women, Betty Ford and Happy Rockefeller, the number of women seeking screening examinations for breast cancer increased dramatically. A similar event involving cervical cancer could result in a surge in screening in both experimen-

*Although the funding period is 3 years, 4 years are included in the measure since census and laboratory data are on a calendar year basis and the program is on a fiscal year.

tal and comparison counties. It should be fairly easy to pinpoint such an event. It would be hoped, however, that the rise in screening in experimental counties would be greater than the rise in comparison counties because of the removal of financial barriers to screening for low-income women in the experimental counties.

A second, more difficult-to-manage threat to internal validity arises from a possible instrumentation effect. It can be anticipated that laboratories supplying the information on the number of Pap smears done each year will get better at gathering that data over the term of the project, which would result in an increase in reported Pap smears in some cases and possibly a decrease in others. Since there is no way to prevent laboratories from knowing whether they are in experimental or comparison counties, it is difficult to predict the effect this might have on data collection. This factor may necessitate periodic reevaluation of the reliability of the measuring instrument.

The other side of controlling for threats to validity arising from "plausible rival hypotheses" is to accumulate as much evidence as possible in support of the primary hypothesis. The multiple time-series design has the advantage of demonstrating the experimental effect in two ways: against the comparison group and against the pretreatment values. The multiple time-series design itself does not control for external threats to validity primarily because of the lack of randomization. These factors will be discussed in the section on generalizability of results.

Data collection procedures. During the planning phase of the project, letters were sent to all members of the Washington State Pathology Society requesting information on the number of Pap smears done each year for the years 1972, 1973, and 1974. These letters went out over the signature of the Society president. Several months later, follow-up letters were sent to nonrespondents. In the seven experimental counties, local pathologists and other physicians were interviewed to identify all the laboratories involved in reading Pap smears for those counties and as a result, several out-of-state laboratories were also surveyed. Following this, a cytotechnologist was employed to make site visits to the local laboratories in the experimental counties and review the relevant laboratory records to check the reliability of written reports. All but one laboratory cooperated with this approach. The pathologist in that laboratory felt that the number of Pap smears he read was "confidential information." Other pathologists in the same area suggested that he did very few Pap smears.

The same data collection procedures will be employed in the comparison counties, that is, interviews with providers to identify sources of cytologic services and a site visit by a cytotechnologist to review records. For the sake of consistency we hope to be able to hire the same cytotechnologist again.

The observation for 1975, 1976, 1977, and 1978 will be gathered by letter each year. It will be necessary to periodically review the providers in each county to keep current with additions and deletions of laboratories.

Matching comparison counties. As in the case of the experimental counties, the comparison counties will be selected in part on the basis of demographic factors associated with risk for cervical cancer. These factors are percent of minorities in the population and percent of families with incomes at or below poverty levels. In addition, the counties will also be matched as urban or rural, using the census definition of an SMSA (Standard Metropolitan Statistical Area) and on total population size.

Strength of the instrument. As noted earlier, the instrument being employed to assess the impact of the screening program on the level of Pap screening in the experimental in contrast to the comparison counties is a survey of laboratories providing cytology services in those counties to ascertain the number of Pap smears done each year. This number will then be compared to the number of women in the county who are age 16 or older. Since two methods of gathering the information are being utilized—written requests for information to the laboratories and cytotechnical review of records—the congruence reliability of the instrument can be evaluated by the correlation between the two measures.

The validity of the instrument will be more difficult to evaluate. Content validity is supported by interviews with local health care providers to identify all the laboratories involved in providing cytologic services for the county. This approach is more acceptable in areas with lower populations such as the six rural counties involved in this program. In the one larger urban county it may be possible to assess the strength of the convergent validity of the instrument by comparison to a random sample survey done in 1974 which presents the percent of women who report having had a Pap smear in the previous 18 months. Data adjustment will be necessary to compare the number of Pap smears reported by laboratories to the percent of women who report having had Pap smears, since the time period of the random sample survey is 18 months compared to 12 months for the laboratory survey and since the random sample survey was administered only to female heads-of-household over age 21. However, a significant level of agreement between these two means of estimating the percentages of women obtaining Pap smears should increase confidence in the validity of the instrument being used in the CCSP evaluation to assess impact.

Another factor continues to potentially threaten the validity of the instrument. Patterns for seeking care vary between the counties. In some areas, community people report that some local people go to other counties for health care, or even to Canada in the case of two experimental counties on the Canadian border. Community people also report that people from outside the county often utilize local providers. The survey of laboratories cannot control for residence of the women whose Pap smears are sent to a particular laboratory. It may be difficult to justify the expense, but a small random survey of the residence of women whose Pap smears are read in various laboratories could give a basis for an adjustment factor to apply to reported members of Pap smears from each laboratory. The assumption would be made that X per cent of the Pap smears read by the laboratory were done on out-of-county women and that X per cent of the women in a particular county went out of county for Pap smears.

It is most likely that given the cost, time, and administrative constraints under which this evaluation will be carried out that the evaluators will rely primarily on the content validity of the measure. That is, the agreement by local health practitioners that the reported number of Pap smears and the laboratories surveyed are a reasonable estimate of the level of Pap smear screening in their counties.

Since the screening program is directed at only one segment of the county's population, low-income women, and the instrument will be measuring screening for the entire population, it is likely that the measurement of program impact will be muted. The question being asked is whether the instrument will be sensitive enough to pick up changes in the level of screening in a subsection of the total population of a county. It

Table A. Data available for multiple time-series analysis

	1972	1973	1974	X	1975	1976	1977	1978	X_0
Experimental counties	O_1	O_2	O_3		O_4	O_5	O_6	O_7	
Comparison counties	O_8	O_9	O_{10}		O_{11}	O_{12}	O_{13}	O_{14}	

is anticipated that the time-series approach with seven observations at yearly intervals will be sufficient to register changes in the level of screening. If evaluation results indicate support for the null hypothesis of no difference, the question of sensitivity of the instrument will remain unanswered.

Cost of carrying out the evaluation. The evaluation will be carried out by the State Office of Research and Planning. They estimate a cost of about $1500 for the first year. In addition, the CCSP will employ a cytotechnologist to complete the gathering of the preprogram data in the comparison counties. Total salary and travel for this aspect will cost about $250.

Analyzing the data from the multiple time-series analysis. The data that will be available at the end of the program are diagrammed in Table A. "O" will be a ratio, the number of Pap smears reported in a county for that year over the number of women age 16 and older in that year; "X" represents the point of the treatment intervention; "X_0" represents the end of the treatment.

As noted earlier, the multiple time-series will give two means for evaluating the impact of the program. The first is by means of pre- and post-treatment values to ascertain whether or not a significant increase in the level of Pap smear screening occurred. The second is by means of comparison to matched counties without the program to demonstrate that the treatment intervention was responsible for any noted changes in the level of screening.

If the screening program has a significant impact on the number of women receiving Pap smears in the experimental counties, this will be noted as a change in both intercept and slope in Fig. A, without a corresponding change or without a change of the same degree for the comparison counties. Campbell and Stanley[17] suggest that the analysis of multiple time-series data to determine the significance of the changes can be done by means of a t test as presented by Mood.[18] To compare the pre- and post-treatment values, a regression is run on the pre-treatment observations (O_1 to O_3 and O_8

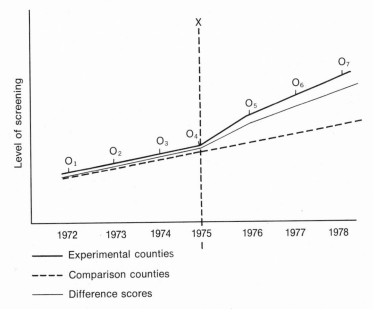

Fig. A. Predicted impact of the CCSP on the level of Pap screening in experimental and comparison counties.

to O_{10}) and a confidence interval is computed. A t test is then used to measure if the change in the intercept exceeds the confidence interval. If it does, it is possible to conclude that the program has made a statistically significant difference. To evaluate the impact of screening in the experimental counties in contrast to the comparison counties, the difference scores at each observation point can be computed (see Fig. A) and analyzed in the same way as the pre- and post-treatment data. Alternatively, analysis of variance can be employed in which the scores of each experimental county are compared with the scores of each control county for the different years.

Generalizability of the results. As with most quasi-experimental designs, the generalizability of the outcome is dependent on the extent to which external threats to validity can be controlled for. In this particular application of a multiple time-series analysis, an interaction between testing and treatment is not a problem because of the independence of the two. An interaction between selection and treatment would also not be a problem because the program is directed toward a very specific population, namely, low-income women. Reactive arrangements are also unlikely to be a problem. The group to whom the treatment will be applied, low-income women, will certainly not be influenced by pretesting. Surveying the laboratories has this advantage over surveying women to ascertain the pretreatment level of screening. The utilization of local resources for education and screening will also reduce the likelihood of a reactive arrangement.

One central and very critical problem exists which will limit generalized application of the treatment. It will be very difficult to really specify what the treatment is, beyond stating the removal of financial barriers to screening and the utilization of county units of the Cancer Society using stated techniques to educate and motivate the target population. The orientation, priorities, and sophistication of local units of the ACS will vary considerably over the country. Thus, if the program in Washington is considered successful, we will at best be able to encourage other areas to attempt a similar model and specify by means of process evaluation particular aspects of the program which were more or less effective. Successful replication of the model in other states will give support to its general usage.

References

1. Boyes, D. A.: The British Columbia screening program, Obstet. Gynecol. Surv. **24:** 1005-1011, 1969.
2. Boyes, D. A.: Personal communication, 1975.
3. Kinlen, L. J., and Doll, R.: Trends in mortality from cancer of the uterus in Canada and in England and Wales, Br. J. Prev. Soc. Med. **27:**146-149, 1973.
4. American Cancer Society: '75 Cancer facts and figures, New York, 1975, The Society.
5. Pedersen, E., Høeg, K., and Kolstad, P.: Mass screening for cancer of the uterine cervix in Østfold County, Norway, Acta Obstet. Gynecol. Scand. supp. 11, 1971.
6. Timonen, S., Nieminen, U., and Kauraniemi, T.: Mass screening for cervical carcinoma in Finland, Ann. Chir. Gynecol. Fenn. **63:**104-112, 1974.
7. Kessner, D. M., Project Director: Contrasts in health status, vol. 2, Washington, D.C., 1973, Institute of Medicine, pp. 192-219.
8. Geller, H.: Probability study of deaths in the next ten years from specific causes, Philadelphia, 1966, Jefferson Medical College.
9. Rochat, R. W.: The prevalence of cervical cancer screening USA: 1970, presented at 1974 annual meeting of American Public Health Association, New Orleans, October, 1974.
10. Alexander, E. E.: Possible etiologies of cancer of the cervix other than *Herpesvirus,* Cancer Res. **33:**1485-1496, 1973.
11. Terris, M., Wilson, F., and Nelson, J.H.: Relationship of circumcision to cancer of the cervix, Proceedings of the Annual Meeting of the American Public Health Association, 1972.
12. Coppleson, M.: The origin and nature of

pre-malignant lesions of the cervix uteri, Int. J. Obstet. Gynecol. 3:539-550, 1970.

13. Wilson, J. M., and Junger, G.: Principles and practice of screening for disease, Geneva, 1968, World Health Organization.

14. Schweitzer, S. O.: Cost effectiveness of early detection of disease, Health Services Research, Spring, 1974.

15. Suchman, E. A.: Evaluative research: principles and practice in public service and social action programs, New York, 1967, Russell Sage Foundation.

16. Williams, W.: Implementation analysis and assessment, Policy Analysis 1:531-566, 1975.

17. Campbell, D. T., and Stanley, J. C.: Experimental and quasi-experimental designs for research, Skokie, Ill., 1966, Rand McNally & Co.

18. Mood, A. Mc.: Introduction to the theory of statistics, New York, 1950, McGraw-Hill Book Co.